Humor as Survival Training for a Stressed-Out World

The 7 Humor Habits Program

Paul McGhee

authorHOUSE®

AuthorHouse™
1663 Liberty Drive
Bloomington, IN 47403
www.authorhouse.com
Phone: 1-800-839-8640

First published by AuthorHouse 7/13/2010

ISBN: 978-1-4520-2183-6 (e)
ISBN: 978-1-4520-2181-2 (sc)

Library of Congress Control Number: 2010909502

Printed in the United States of America
Bloomington, Indiana

This book is printed on acid-free paper.

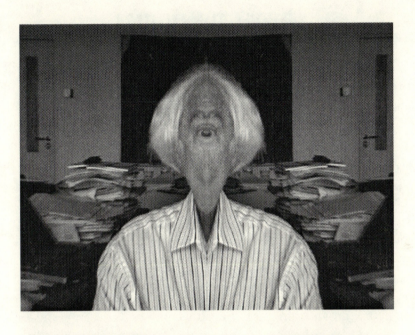

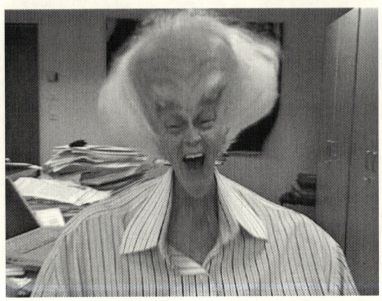

About the Author

Paul McGhee, PhD, is a psychologist, and is one of the world's foremost authorities on the benefits of building more humor and laughter into your life. He is internationally known for his own humor research, having spent 20 years conducting research on humor and laughter while teaching at the university level. He has published a dozen books on humor, along with many scientific articles on the topic. The effectiveness of the 7 Humor Habits (7HH) Program, presented in this book, has been documented on three continents. It is the first book to present a research-based program for boosting your sense of humor.

Dr. McGhee has worked full time as a professional speaker for the past 15 years. He has given talks on humor in 11 countries. His keynotes are most often for corporate and healthcare organizations, but he also provides programs for early childhood educators and senior citizens. He is at the cutting edge of the current movement to bring a lighter attitude to the workplace, while maintaining high standards of competence and professionalism. His programs most commonly focus on how keeping your sense of humor provides the emotional resilience required to work effectively (and provide quality care in hospitals) in the midst of mounting work demands and job-related stress. Workshops focus on learning to use humor to cope with stress.

To learn more about the health and coping benefits of humor, and to obtain more information about his programs, see his website, www.LaughterRemedy.com.

Dr. McGhee's work has been featured in *The New York Times*, *USA Today*, *Newsweek*, *Scientific American Mind*, *GEO* (in Europe), and many other American and European magazines and newspapers. He has also been featured on the *Learning Channel*, *National Public Radio*, *PBS* television, and many other American and European television and radio programs.

He is President of The Laughter Remedy, in Wilmington, DE. If you would like to arrange for a keynote or workshop by Dr. McGhee for your organization, see his website for contact information.

CONTENTS

Introduction

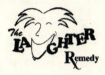

How do you make God laugh? Make plans.

"A person without a sense of humor is like a wagon without springs—jolted by every pebble in the road."

(Henry Ward Beecher)

In the year in which this book was published (2010), the United States found itself caught in the grips of the second year of the greatest economic crisis the country has faced since the Great Depression of the 1930s. Even before the financial meltdown of late 2008, we were faced with constantly escalating job demands, crippling increases in healthcare costs, mounting challenges to raising a family with shrinking financial resources, a war that seemed to have no end in sight, and the continued threat of terrorism. Across the country—and in many other countries, as well—people's coping skills have been pushed to their limits. More than ever before, we all need special skills that give us the emotional resilience we need to survive in an increasingly stressed-out world. Your sense of humor is one set of skills that are essential to meeting the challenges to your emotional survival that you're sure to encounter in the days and years ahead. This book shows you how to develop the basic Humor Habits required to use your sense of humor to cope.

Individuals and small groups have been using the approach presented in this book to learn to use humor to cope with the stress in their lives for the past 14 years. While many people know from their own experience that it works, numerous studies have also now documented the effectiveness of this program in the USA, Austria, Switzerland, Germany and Australia. It will also work for you; all you have to do is put in some time and energy and fun into it for eight weeks in order to build up the humor habits discussed here to the point that they help you cope with the stress in your life.

Why Make the Effort to Improve Your Sense of Humor?

If you're lucky, you had parents who modeled a good sense of humor as you were growing up. They knew that a good sense of humor is just like the shock absorber on your car. It smoothes out the bumpy spots in the road of life and helps you keep moving to your destination without getting stuck in every rut in the road.

Physical Health Benefits

The companion to this book, *Humor: The Lighter Path to Resilience and Health* (2010) provides the answer to why it is worth the effort (and the fun that goes with it) that you'll spend improving your sense of humor using the 7 Humor Habits Training Program (referred to throughout the book as the 7HH Program) provided here. That book discusses the latest research on the many physical and mental/emotional health benefits resulting from humor and laughter. These benefits include such general health promoting mechanisms as a stronger immune system, reduced blood levels of stress hormones, and pain reduction, as well as documented health benefits in connection with specific diseases—including coronary heart disease, asthma, chronic obstructive pulmonary disorder (COPD), arthritis, skin allergies and diabetes.

The specific mechanisms responsible for improvement of these diseases are still not well understood, but reduced levels of damaging stress hormones, enhancement of the immune system, and reduced levels of damaging cytokines explain some of the benefits. One thing is certainly clear: humor's capacity to generate positive emotion and substitute a positive emotion for a negative one when you're angry, anxious or depressed, plays a key role in all of the health benefits provided by humor.

Using Humor to Cope with Stress

There is an enormous body of evidence (also discussed in *Humor: The Lighter Path to Resilience and Health*) that your sense of humor is a powerfully ally in helping you cope with any form of life stress. Stress is now reaching epidemic levels among people at all socioeconomic levels. If you're lucky enough to still have a job, you know that job stress has increased in recent years. The past 15 years, however, have witnessed a (slowly) growing number of North American companies which are learning to put humor and fun to work—and this increase is clearly a result of their realization of the need to find effective tools to help employees manage mounting job stress. Humor is recognized as a skill which can help sustain a healthy bottom line. Emotional intelligence is increasingly viewed as being crucial to any successful organization, and the use of humor to manage one's own emotions and the emotions of others is a key component of emotional intelligence.

Growing Interest in Improving One's Sense of Humor

As awareness of the many benefits of humor has grown, so has interest in developing the skills required to obtain those benefits. Patients coping with serious illnesses (or recovering from serious injuries), stressed-out employees, managers who want to communicate more effectively or boost productivity, parents trying to cope with the modern challenge of raising kids, self-help and support groups, individuals interested in personal growth—all want to learn to lighten up. Even counselors and psychotherapists are now giving a serious look at humor as a coping skill for their patients. The rapidly growing number of "therapeutic laughter" or "laughter yoga" groups across the USA and in many other countries is another reflection of this growing interest in reaping humor's rewards.

"A man will confess to treason, murder, arson, false teeth, or a wig. How many of them will own up to a lack of humor?"

(Frank Moore Colby)

I made a presentation in Philadelphia in 2009 at the First World Congress of the International Positive Psychology Association. That presentation was based on an assessment of the effectiveness of the 7HH Program presented in this book. That particular study was completed in Switzerland. About 40% of the people attending this conference were from countries other than the USA. From 11 a.m. until 5 p.m., I had a non-stop stream of people stopping by to discuss the poster presenting the results of the study. In 25 years of attending similar conferences, I had never before seen such widespread international interest in a single poster presentation. The consistent feedback I got was that this kind of program was sorely needed in their country, and that nothing like this existed. Several inquired about how to go about making a translation of the Program available in their country.

Who is the 7 Humor Habits Program Designed for?

This book focuses on seven habits that are essential to developing a well-rounded sense of humor—a sense of humor which will help you cope with the mounting stress on your job and elsewhere in your life, and make a significant contribution to your daily happiness and success at work. No other book offers such a detailed path in showing what you need to do to develop these habits and skills and have access to them in your daily life.

The 7HH Program is especially designed for the humor impaired, but you'll still benefit if you already have a good sense of humor. Consider yourself humor impaired only if you've forgotten how—or never learned—to enjoy and produce humor. Many people who never used to be humor impaired have become so precisely because of the mounting stress in their lives. These are people who have lost their ability to lighten up and be playful, even when everyone else around them is doing so. I often see people in my programs who say to me, "You know, I used to have a great sense of humor. I used to be the one who always saw the light side of things. But somewhere along the way, I lost it . . ." These people have succumbed to what I call TS—Terminal Seriousness.

If this sounds like you, or someone you love, you need to realize that TS is a killer. It kills the quality of your life! It kills the sense of aliveness, joy, and fun in your life. In this sense, it is similar to suffering from clinical depression. It can even kill your effectiveness on your job, because it sets you up for extra stress—both at work and in your personal life. It is this mounting job stress, relationship problems, health and financial problems, terrorist threats, and more, which has increased the number of people now suffering from TS. Luckily, however, it's not a permanent condition. By spending a week or two on each of the Seven Humor Habits discussed in this book, you can pull yourself up by your emotional bootstraps and forever escape any future vulnerability to TS.

We generally assume that it's the serious employee who is most effective on the job. But let's consider two equally competent employees doing the same job, and who have comparable levels of motivation to do their jobs well. And let's further assume that they have comparable high levels of stress built into their job. The one with TS will generally be less effective—not more—in his/her work in the long run. Why? Because s/he is likely to be more vulnerable to stress, experience more burnout, and suffer from lower levels of job satisfaction and morale. S/he will be less resilient in the face of ever-growing job demands, unpredictable crises, and the uncertainty of permanent employment. S/he will be less happy on the job, and experience lower levels of the intrinsic pleasure in the work s/he's paid to do. Having a good sense of humor helps turn all of these negatives into a positive (or at least a weaker negative).

Many of us have been so serious for so long that we've acquired another unwanted condition. I call it AADS—Acquired Amusement Deficiency Syndrome. AADS destroys your sense of joy and aliveness and sets you up for a persistent negative mood as daily hassles and problems accumulate.

If you're suffering from AADS, you need an attitude adjustment. That's why the 7HH Program starts by helping you learn to adopt a more playful attitude, both on your job and in your relationships. This does not mean that you're to stop taking your job and relationships seriously; in fact, it is precisely because they are important to you that you want to learn to lighten up in dealing with them. Learning to become more playful and poke fun at both your relationships and your job will increase your satisfaction and effectiveness in both.

How to be Sure this Book Works for You

This book is not designed to make you a stand-up comedian, although you will improve your joke-telling and other comedic skills. It is also not a book of comedy-writing techniques, although you will have many opportunities to create your own humor, and will become more skilled at doing so. The goal of the book is to improve your sense of humor to the point that it does not abandon you when you're having a bad day! It teaches you how to use your sense of humor to cope with the stress in your life. And it does this by building up some basic humor habits on your good days.

Most people who attend my humor seminars around the country want to learn what they can do starting *right now* to use humor to cope with their stress-filled lives. Unfortunately, that's not the way it works. Your sense of humor will always abandon you when something makes you upset, anxious, or depressed—unless you develop some basic humor skills and habits first, when you're not under stress. This book shows you how to do just that, in a step-by-step fashion.

You can use this book either by yourself, with a partner or as part of a group that is meeting regularly to learn to improve their sense of humor. The Program always has more impact if you have at least one other person (your spouse, a friend, a colleague at work, etc.) who is going through it with you. Home Play is provided for each humor habit. That is, suggestions are made of things to do over a one- or two-week period that will help develop the skills associated with each habit. As you would expect, people who actually do more of the Home Play make more progress. So what you get out of this book depends totally on the skill-building effort you put into it. But don't approach this as work! You are guaranteed to have more fun in your daily life as you practice each of these healthy humor habits.

The Humor Habits

The First Habit you are asked to strengthen is the habit of building more humor into your daily life. While doing this, you are offered guidelines for better understanding your current sense of humor. You will gain an initial understanding of your current humor strengths and weakness, as well as the influences that produced them. You will take a sense of humor pre-test (included at the back of this book) at this point, so that you can later compare it to the post-test you'll take after finishing the Program and determine how much you've gained.

The Second Humor Habit you'll develop does not involve humor *per se*, but is actually the key to your success in the rest of the Program. It involves simply cultivating a playful attitude within yourself, so that you have access to this attitude when you need it. This is the basic foundation out of which your own natural sense of humor emerges. Humor is actually a form of mental play, so when you become more comfortable with being playful in general, your mind is just naturally more ready to find and enjoy humor. Every great comedian has immediate access to this playful attitude toward life, even if they have a "dry" sense of humor.

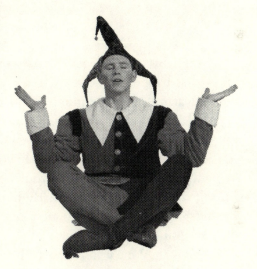

It's all a matter of practicing the humor habits. Meditation won't do it!

The Third Humor Habit is to laugh more often and more heartily than you usually do. Again, this is not a humor skill; it is more a matter of emotional expression. It is included here because there is good reason to believe that some of the health and coping benefits of humor may well come from the physical act of laughter, and there are many who read this book who—either because of their temperament or past personal experiences—are simply not very good at real belly laughter.

Humor Habit number four is the first true humor habit you'll work on—learning to play with language. You'll first build your skill at telling memorized jokes and funny stories. This will start tuning you in on the different techniques that are involved in verbal humor, giving special attention to puns. You will then start building the habit of creating your own spontaneous verbal humor.

A guy walks into a fancy bar, but they won't let him in without a necktie. So he gets his jumper cables out of his car and ties them around his neck. He goes back to the bar and says, "OK, can I get in now?" They answer, "Well, all right, but you better not start anything."

The Fifth Humor Habit focuses on finding a light side of the things that happen in your own everyday life. This is an essential skill for learning to use humor to manage stress. You'll see that you're surrounded by opportunities for humor every day, but just have not seen them. You'll learn how to see funny and think funny.

The Sixth Humor Habit builds up your ability to laugh at yourself. You will learn to poke fun at your own mistakes and qualities of yourself that you don't particularly like. You'll learn to stop taking yourself so seriously, even though you continue to take your work and responsibilities seriously.

Finally, the Seventh and last Humor Habit focuses on having access to all the habits you've cultivated to this points when you're having a bad day. So this habit asks you to work on applying your abilities to create verbal humor, find humor in everyday situations and poke fun at yourself in the midst of stressful situations in your life. Equally important, of course, is the habit of generating that basic playful attitude within yourself when you're under stress. If you have done a good percentage of the Home Play to this point, you will already have begun to make progress in having access to your sense of humor in situations where it used to abandon you.

The final week or two of the Program asks you to make an effort to "put it all together," integrating all the skills and habits developed in the program so that you can readily move from one habit to another spontaneously. Since you will have been focusing on one habit at a time to this point, you may have lost some of the gains from the earlier ones as you shifted your attention to later ones. To build all the habits into a permanent part of your personality, you need a week or two concentrating on all of them at once.

While you can spend as little as one week cultivating each habit, the benefits you receive will go up sharply if you spend two weeks on each. You will also benefit more by having a partner who goes through the Program with you (so you have someone to talk to about your experiences while going through the Program).

Your Personal Humor Log

Before beginning the 7HH Program, you will be asked to create in your computer a special file into which you will make written additions as you work on developing skills associated with each humor habit. You can also do this by hand, using a spiral notebook devoted to your efforts in the Program during a two- to four-month period (depending on whether you devote one or two weeks to each habit).

> *"You've got to realize when all goes well, and everything is beautiful, you have no comedy. It's when somebody steps on the bride's train or belches during the ceremony, then you've got comedy."* (Phyllis Diller)

For each humor habit, you will find a section called, "Humor Log: Things to Do and Think About." This section will always include a lengthy list of things for you to think about and questions for you to answer in connection with issues directly related to that particular humor habit. You should be sure to fight the temptation to skip over these Humor Log requests. You may find yourself wanting to just jump right into working on the specific humor activities designed to strengthen that habit. This is a big mistake, since thinking about the important issues raised in connection with each habit in the Humor

Log sections is crucial to strengthening the habit and making it a lasting and integral part of your daily life.

Background Material Introducing each Humor Habit

A general discussion of important issues related to each humor habit is provided before you are asked to complete the Humor Log questions related to that habit; this discussion is designed to enrich your understanding of that particular habit. Be sure to read this material before answering the Humor Log questions, since many of the issues raised by the those questions are discussed there.

The Home Play

At the end of each humor habit "chapter," you will find a list of suggestions of things to do over the course of the following week or two to build or strengthen that particular habit. It is called "Home Play," and not "Homework," because—even though you're making a serious effort to improve your sense of humor—this should be fun!

If you want to improve your sense of humor, you'll have to actively engage your sense of humor. It doesn't matter how many sit coms, comedy films, or *Far Side* and *Dilbert* cartoons you see; you won't get better at using humor to cope unless you start actively generating and finding your own humor. Just as no one ever made it to the Olympics (or Carnegie Hall) by watching others practice, you'll never learn to use humor to cope unless you start making the effort to actively develop your own humor skills. The Home Play shows you the things you need to do to develop the skills associated with each habit.

You are not expected to do all the Home Play provided for each habit. A wide range of suggestions is provided because different individuals will feel more comfortable doing different activities. The important thing is to be actively engaged doing some of the Home Play as you work on each habit. But you don't have to do it all to make good progress with that habit. Still, the more you do, the greater the progress you'll make—and the more rapidly you'll learn to use humor to cope.

Create a "Daily Humor Diary." You will be asked to create a Daily Humor Diary to use on an ongoing basis as you proceed through the 7HH Program. The purpose of this diary is to help you keep track of—and remember—the things you do and observations you make in connection with the Home Play assigned for each humor habit. (It is hereafter simply called a Humor Diary, but the assumption is that you will keep this with you and record things in it every day.) This Diary should be a small notebook (or something comparable) which you can keep with you at all times, in which you record specific funny things you do or see during the day; otherwise, you'll soon forget them. You don't have to discuss the observation in great detail, but be sure to get enough information down that it will later remind you of the details. For important observations related to any habit you're working on, record your observations and ideas in your Humor Log.

In you are going through the Program with others, as part of a group, the Diary will facilitate your discussion of your efforts at the Home Play since your last meeting. If you are going through the Program alone, you will also benefit from keeping the Diary, since it will help you keep particular aspects of the Home Play on the "front burner" for a couple of weeks. It will also increase your awareness of whether you really are making progress in the Program.

Running a Humor Habits Training Group

This book is designed to be used by individuals (although it has more impact if you have a partner going through it at the same time). However, the author's experience with an earlier version of the 7HH Program has made it clear that many organizations are interested in setting up an opportunity for people to go through the program as a small group. This has occurred in churches (one church in Texas has an ongoing Humor Chalice Group that has met for years, continuing to have humor discussions long after completing the Program two times), lunch meetings in corporate settings, support groups, senior retirement communities, and even college courses.

Any group meeting on a regular basis can use the Program, with one of the members leading it all the way through, or a different member leading each session.

At the end of each of the habit chapters, you will find a section called "Group Session." This section offers specific guidelines and topics for discussion, enabling anyone who is comfortable leading groups to lead sessions devoted to the 7 Humor Habits Program.

Including the Program as Part of a College Course

During the past decade, a growing number of college courses have asked students to complete the 7HH Program (as it was represented my earlier book—now out of print—*Health, Healing and the Amuse System*) as part of the course requirements for a course focusing on humor research in general, or more specifically on humor and health. These courses are always popular undergraduate courses. Each professor, naturally, teaches the course as s/he sees fit. However, a general structure that seems to work well is to devote one class per week to the Program (splitting time between discussing the Home Play from the previous meeting and basic concepts and issues related to the humor habit for the coming week). The other two class meetings each week (or one meeting if it is a Tuesday/Thursday course) are devoted to the more substantive content of the course. The Group Session sections of each habit are ideally suited for a college course.

This kind of course works better in a semester system (15 weeks long) than a quarter system (10 weeks long), but can be managed in either. Instructors need to be aware that the timing of the Seventh Humor Habit (Find Humor in the Midst of Stress) may well coincide with high stress levels at the end of the term in a quarter system—a time when term papers and final exams generate sharply increased pressure on students. This makes it a real challenge to demonstrate significant gains between the pre- and post-test in a quarter system.

Feedback from instructors teaching a course like this shows that many students are not expecting the course to be a "serious" (or substantive) course; they're expecting something like a comedy show or the opportunity to watch a lot of sit coms. Nonetheless, students generally get great enjoyment out of the course once they see what it is really about.

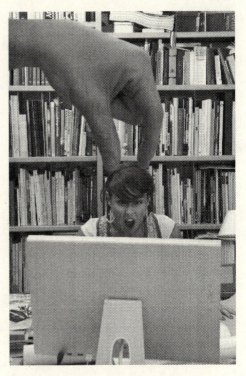

The course also seems to work especially well when the instructor goofs up now and then, making mistakes or otherwise poking fun at him/ herself. As one instructor put it, "It's important for me to make a fool out of myself." This sets the tone and makes it easier for students to enter into the spirit of fun and even poke fun at themselves.

As is recommended here for individuals completing the Program alone, instructors for these courses invariably assign only parts of the Home Play each week. Assigning all of it creates an impossible assignment and takes the fun out of it. Students keep track of their efforts in doing the Home Play assignments in their Humor Diary.

If you are considering teaching a college course on humor, and would like to examine a sample course syllabus developed by one instructor who has taught a course based on the 7HH Program numerous times, see the reference section for Appendix 2 for information on how to contact him for a copy of his current syllabus.

How to Benefit from the Group Session Section if You're Completing the Program Alone

Each "Group Session" section suggests a wide range of topics for discussion related to the habit participants have just been working on. You will receive greater benefits in going through this Program by yourself if you use those discussion suggestions as a source of issues to reflect upon yourself. Just thinking about them boosts your rate of progress through the Program. And your progress will be accelerated even more if you write down your thoughts in your Humor Log. Writing them down clarifies what you think about the issue in question. It will also add to the benefits you receive from the Program.

Research Documenting the Effectiveness of the 7 Humor Habits Program

It may be easier for you to spend two to four months worth of your valuable time and energy going through this Humor Habits Program if you know that it really works. Studies have been completed in several countries demonstrating the effectiveness of the Program for college students, adults of varying ages, and even senior citizens in their 70s. This research is discussed in both summary form and in detail in Appendix 1. Read at least the general summary before beginning the Program.

Assessing Your Progress

You will find in Appendix 3 a "pre-test" and "post-test" of your sense of humor. Separate parts of this measure assess each of the habits in the Program. You will be asked to take the pre-test before beginning the First Habit and to then not look at it again until you have completed the entire Program and the post-test. You can then compare your answers on the pre- and post-test and make your own determination of your progress.

THE FIRST HABIT

SURROUND YOURSELF WITH HUMOR (AND THINK ABOUT THE NATURE OF YOUR SENSE OF HUMOR)

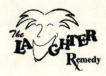

"You show your character in nothing more clearly than by what you think laughable."

(Goethe)

"A person reveals his character by nothing so clearly as the joke he resents."

(G. C. Lichtenberg)

THE FIRST HABIT OF PEOPLE who fully reap the many health and coping benefits offered by humor is daily exposure to humor. They do this in many ways, like watching sit coms on television, going to funny movies, seeking out the cartoons first when they open up a magazine, hanging around funny friends and colleagues, and, of course, initiating their own humor in everyday life. While they don't necessarily do things just to make those around them laugh, they also do not check their sense of humor at the door when they go to work or church—or when they get caught in rush-hour traffic.

You are asked to do two things here. The first is to develop the habit of immersing yourself in humor when the opportunity arises—and when it seems appropriate. Doing this from now on will make it easier for you to stay focused on building specific humor habits later on. (Note: the words "habit" and "skill" will be used interchangeably throughout this book, since most of the habits discussed are based on specific skills that can be practiced and strengthened.) The second is to make an active effort to better understand your sense of humor.

Take the Sense of Humor Pre-Test

Before beginning the 7HH Program, complete the sense of humor pre-test found at the end of the book. This test assesses where you now stand in terms of key dimensions of your sense of humor—especially those related to the 7 Humor Habits. Once you have completed the pre-test, put it away and avoid looking at it again until after you have completed the entire Program. You will then be asked to take the post-test. Comparing your pre- and post-test answers will enable you to determine how much progress you've made.

Immerse Yourself in Humor

If you have a poorly developed sense of humor, or a generally serious demeanor, humor probably has not played a prominent role in your life. The easiest way to start changing that is simply to build more *outside sources* of humor into your daily life. Spend more time around friends who make you laugh. Seek out funny films, TV programs, and comedy DVDs. Look at cartoons in magazines and other publications. Go to comedy clubs. Immerse yourself in humor wherever you can find it. This will not only be fun, but will also help you better understand your own sense of humor as you begin to actively reflect on your reactions to different kinds of humor. It will also add a more positive, playful focus to your everyday interactions with people and ease you into noticing more humor in your own life. It will whet your appetite to start building up your humor skills.

> *"A man will confess to treason, murder, arson, false teeth, or a wig. How many of them will own up to a lack of humor?"*
>
> (Frank Moore Colby)

"You've got to realize when all goes well, and everything is beautiful, you have no comedy. It's when somebody steps on the bride's train or belches during the ceremony, then you've got comedy."

(Phyllis Diller)

The Humor Log exercises provide guidelines for using this increased exposure to get a better picture of your sense of humor. This initial extra immersion in to humor is much more important than you might think. It will help build a foundation for creating your own humor later on. So be sure to fight any tendency to skip over working to cultivate the First Habit.

Humor Log: Things to Do and Think About

This first set of Humor Log exercises is designed to help you begin to understand your current sense of humor and how it has developed the way it has during your life.

Nature or Your Current Sense of Humor

Use the exercises provided below to map out your own humor profile. Record your responses in your own personal Humor Log.

1. List your current favorite sit coms on television.
2. List the comedy films you enjoyed the most in the last decade. Who made you laugh the most in these films?
3. List the stand-up comedians who you think are very funny. Put a star next to the three you like the most.
4. List the comedians who turn you off (because you find their humor distasteful, boring, sexist, or unoriginal, etc.).
5. What are your favorite cartoons in magazines and newspapers?
6. Among your friends and colleagues, who do you find funny? Who always makes you laugh?

7. What kinds of everyday situations do you laugh at most often?
8. Record in your Humor Log any common threads you see in your humor preferences.
9. Based on all the above, describe your sense of humor.

"In matters of humor, what is appealing to one person is appalling to another." (Melvin Helitzer)

Nature of Your Sense of Humor while Growing Up

One of the best ways to improve your understanding of your present sense of humor is to examine its development during your childhood and adolescence, including the impact of your parents and other significant figures. Record your responses to the following questions in your Humor Log.

1. Were you a funny kid? Were you generally playful or serious?
2. Describe the way you remember your sense of humor as a child. (If your parents are living, talk to them about what you were like as a kid. Specifically ask if you laughed more/less than other kids, told a lot of riddles and jokes, played practical jokes, etc. You may be surprised to find that their memory of this does not match your own.)
3. Were you a funny adolescent or young adult? Describe the way you remember your sense of humor during adolescence and early adulthood.
4. Use the 4-point scale shown below to rate these five basic ways of showing a good sense of humor. Do so for A) the elementary school years, B) adolescence, and C) your early adult years.

	Child.	Adol.	Adult
1 = Very typical of me		2 = Somewhat typical of me	
3 = Not very typical of me		4 = Not at all typical of me	
Enjoyment of others' humor	_____	_____	_____
Initiation of humor	_____	_____	_____
Finding humor in daily life	_____	_____	_____
Laughing at yourself	_____	_____	_____
Finding humor under stress	_____	_____	_____

Based on these ratings, record in your Humor Log how your sense of humor has changed over time. If you're middle-aged or older, also look at your sense of humor throughout your adult years.

Early Influences on Your Sense of Humor

Record your answers in your Humor Log.

1) Who, during your childhood, adolescence, and early adulthood years, had the greatest influence (positive and negative) on the development of your sense of humor?
2) Describe your mother's sense of humor.
3) Describe your father's sense of humor.
4) What similarities do you see between your parents' sense of humor and your own?
5) How did your mother influence your sense of humor?
6) How did your father influence your sense of humor?
7) How did other people (grandparents, uncles/aunts, neighbors, etc.) influence your sense of humor?

Did your parents show a sense of humor with each other? With you? In the way they handled everyday problems? Can you remember them having a generally playful style of interaction with you during your childhood? Were they humor initiators? Did they laugh out loud a lot? Could they laugh at themselves? Did they react positively when you made an effort to do something funny (e.g., by going along with your riddles)? Ask yourself the same questions about grandparents or other significant figures in your life.

Be sure to include negative parental reactions to your early attempts at humor. Some parents feel that humor and play create bad habits that will interfere with the ability to get a good education, get a job, etc. They feel they're doing their children a favor by forcing them to get serious about life early. In fact, they're robbing their children of a powerful coping skill. Look for continuity in the nature of your sense of humor over the years, or for points at which it took a sudden step forward or backward. It may have blossomed in childhood only to gradually disappear into the woodwork of your personality during adulthood. Or perhaps it first emerged in adolescence or adulthood.

Current Influences on Your Sense of Humor

Record your answers in your Humor Log.

1) In what situations does your sense of humor now show up most often? Think about when and where you laugh the most and initiate the most humor. Is it at work? At home? What is it about these situations that brings out your sense of humor? Think about both the nature of the situation and the people who are there.

2) In what situations does your sense of humor now show up least often? Are there any situations (at work, home, or elsewhere) in which you are always serious? What is it about these situations that causes your sense of humor to abandon you? Think about both the people present and the situation itself.

3) Do you show more of a sense of humor with men or with women? Why? Think about this both in terms of whether (and how often) you initiate humor and how you react to the humor of others.

GROUP SESSION

Use this first group session to talk about participants' goals in completing the 7 Humor Habits Program, along with any other issues pertinent to your particular group. Also discuss as many of the exercises and questions presented in the Humor Log Exercises as time permits. Do this for all future meetings, as well.

The group leader should decide whether topics are to be discussed in pairs, groups of 3, 4, etc., or among the group as a whole. The most effective approach is often to first discuss a topic in pairs, allowing each person in the group a chance to talk, and then open it up to the group as a whole.

Introductions

If some members of the group do not know each other, find a playful way to allow people to introduce themselves. For example, each person can give their name and produce a silly sound or action that expresses how they felt when they walked into the room. Or they can briefly describe the silliest, funniest, or most embarrassing thing they ever did.

Goals You Want to Achieve

Each participant should pair up with another person and describe what s/he would like to gain from the Program. For example, which aspects of their sense of humor would they especially like to improve? If the group is small, goals may be described to the whole group.

Opening Fun Activity

Start each meeting with some kind of fun activity to help put the group into a more playful mood. This should be a game which invites cooperation and draws people together in some form of playful— even silly—interaction, not a competitive game. The leader can have something prepared for the first session, but a volunteer should be asked to bring in a fun activity for each of the remaining sessions.

Feel free to play your favorite games from childhood, since they are usually very effective in regenerating the playful mental attitude that nurtures your sense of humor.

What is Humor?

You know when something is funny to you, but have you ever thought about how you would define humor? Ask for a few definitions from the group and see if there's a consensus. What does it mean to say that you have a sense of humor? What do you really mean when you say something is funny?

Humor Terms

Break into small groups and generate as many words as you can which relate to humor and laughter in some way. For example, you might include funny, incongruous, bizarre, sarcastic, etc. There are many more. Develop as big a list as you can, and think about the meaning of these terms. This exercise will help you map out the distinctions we make about humor.

Describe Your Sense of Humor

Describe your sense of humor to a partner, using whatever terms come to mind. Also discuss the following if time permits:

1) What medium of humor do you prefer (films, stand-up comedy, cartoons in magazines or books, literature, sit coms, etc.)?
2) What are your favorite sit coms, comedy films, stand-up comedians, or (print) cartoons? Why do you like them?
3) What kind of humor do you dislike, or find distasteful? Why do you dislike it? Is it annoying to find others laughing at humor you find distasteful?

Analysis of Particular Examples of Humor

Use a few specific jokes or cartoons to generate a discussion of why group members do or do not find them funny. One of the jokes or cartoons should be put-down humor. Does one's reaction to such jokes depend on their attitude toward, or liking of, the person or idea disparaged? Use this as a vehicle for discussing your views about put-down humor in general. Why is disparagement humor so popular? Why do most countries have a favorite victim in jokes? Is political humor generally of the put-down variety? Can you laugh at jokes disparaging others without really disparaging them?

Influences on Your Sense of Humor

Use specific questions from the Humor Log exercises to discuss with a partner the most important influences on your sense of humor, including both past and present influences.

Sex Differences

What gender differences have you observed in humor? Do these differences also occur in other cultures or subcultures? Make it a point to discuss stereotypes.

Visualization Exercise

Think back to a period of your childhood when you had a lot of joy and laughter. Relive in your mind's eye a specific instance when you were having fun and laughing. Recapture what led up to the situation, who was there, and how you felt. Be with the experience for a couple of minutes. Then think about whether you still have experiences like that today. Discuss the feelings you experienced during this exercise.

The Negative Side of Humor

This Humor Habits Program focuses on achieving the many positive benefits resulting from humor, but humor can also take negative forms and trigger negative outcomes. Discuss any of the negative aspects of humor that you can think of. Some possibilities include 1) judgments by colleagues that you're unprofessional, incompetent, immature or not serious about your work, 2) people who are always joking when you're trying to have a serious conversation, 3) insensitivity to the appropriate time or place for humor, 4) offensive forms of humor, and 5) people who laugh indiscriminately at everything.

Is it too Late to Improve Your Sense of Humor?

Many people think that you're either born with a good sense of humor, or you're not—and there's not much you can do about it. Do you agree with this? Are you too old to improve your sense of humor? Are your parents too old? Is it ever too late to learn to lighten up? Why do some people come out of their "mid-life crisis" with a lighter attitude toward their work, and toward life generally?

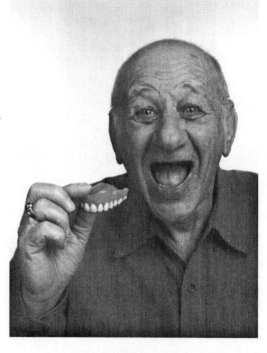

Hey, it's funny to me!
That's good enough.

Choose Telephone Partners

You will make greater progress in improving your sense of humor if you have a regular opportunity to talk to someone else about your efforts at each step. Organize telephone teams (two or three people per team). Agree to call each other at least once between sessions to discuss how you're doing. This will help sustain your motivation to keep doing the Home Play, and will add to the fun you have along the way.

Home Play

[Note: You will almost certainly find that the Home Play associated with each of the 7 Humor Habits includes more than you can possibly do during the week or two you devote to strengthening each habit. This is by design, since different people will feel more comfortable with different Home Play suggestions. *So it is not essential that you do all of the Home Play, but you must do some of it.* One option is to focus your efforts on one of the Home Play activities each day. Choose the suggestions that appeal to you the most. Or focus on areas that you consider personal weaknesses. The important thing is to be actively engaged with some aspect of the Home Play throughout the week. Obviously, the more you do, the more progress you'll make.

Remember to keep a Humor Diary, documenting what you're doing in connection with the Home Play, your observations, insights, etc. This will be especially helpful in enabling you to pull up details if you're going to be discussing the First Habit with a group in a week or so.]

1) Do the Humor Log exercises. Record your responses in your notebook or computer.
2) Make it a point to seek out humor from some professional source each day. This might include sit coms or other comedy programs on television, comedy films (in a theater or at home), books of cartoons, magazine and newspaper cartoons, CDs of stand-up comedians, etc.
3) If you spend a lot of time in your car (e.g., driving to work), collect comedy CDs (many libraries have a good supply of these) and spend some time listening to comedians each day.
4) As you listen to comedy CDs, or think about your favorite comedians, make it a point to think about their humor styles. Which aspects of each comedian's style seem to fit your personality and sense of humor? Consider copying these comedians in any way that feels comfortable as you work on developing your own sense of humor.
5) Find at least one print cartoon each week that has some special significance for you, or which you find especially funny, and

put it in a high visibility place at work (e.g., on your desk, or on a bulletin board) or at home (e.g., on the refrigerator). Be on the lookout for cartoons you like, and add regularly to your collection. If you find yourself with too many, put the old ones in a folder and save them as you replace them with new ones. You may want to create a booklet of your favorite cartoons that you can look at whenever you need a good laugh.

6) Read one funny novel.

7) Go to your local bookstore (or library) and look through several cartoon books. Buy (or borrow) the one you like the most.

8) Find a library that has comedy CDs and sign out several. Listen to one every day. If you have a CD player in your car, ideal times to do this are on the way to and from work. If you jog or take walks, listen to the CDs as you do so. When possible, find a time when you can listen without distraction. Notice the effect this has on your mood. Make note of this effect in your Humor Diary.

9) Go to one comedy film or watch a comedy DVD.

10) Watch several sit coms and decide which programs you like the best. Use these as a basis for thinking about your own sense of humor.

11) Get a joke book and read through it.

12) Think about the nature of your sense of humor, and about influences on the development of your sense of humor. Talk to people who know you well about how they view your sense of humor. Develop a clear view of the strong and weak aspects of your sense of humor. Jot down notes related to this in your Humor Diary as ideas occur to you; then write down your conclusions in your Humor Log before moving on to the next habit.

The Second Habit

Cultivate a Playful Attitude

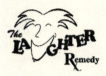

"The human need to play is a powerful one. When we ignore it, we feel there is something missing in our lives."

(Leo Buscaglia)

"So long as there's a bit of a laugh going, things are all right. As soon as this infernal seriousness, like a grassy sea, heaves up, everything is lost."

(D. H. Lawrence)

IF YOU HAVE AN INCURABLE disease, doctors say that you have a terminal illness. The disease has progressed to the point that only a miracle could help you recover. Some people have been so serious and somber for so long that it seems hopeless for them to ever again show a sense of joy, aliveness and fun in life. They are suffering from a condition I call "terminal seriousness," or simply TS.

Of course, it is appropriate to be serious in many situations—including most of the time at work. I'm not suggesting here that you should never be serious. My concern is for people who are always serious. The problem arises when you lose the capacity to be playful—when you are unable to lighten up even when the situation calls for it.

"Life is too serious to be taken seriously." (Oscar Wilde)

15

The key to the Second Habit is the realization that you can take your job, terrorism, cancer, the country's (and your own) financial problems and any other difficult circumstance seriously, but still take yourself lightly. You can maintain your commitment to act to change the problems you see without being a deadly serious person all the time. When you learn this, you'll be amazed by the impact it has on the quality of your life.

The Basic Foundation for Your Sense of Humor

The key to getting started in improving your sense of humor is the rediscovery of the playful attitude you had when you were a child. Children are, by nature, playful. They would spend all day playing if you let them. The joyous laughter that accompanies their play leaves no doubt that they are happy. However, while all parents want their children to be happy, they also want them to become responsible adults and to make something of their lives. And many view play as an obstacle to personal achievement. They feel that the sooner they get their kids to stop playing and get serious about life, the greater their chances of later becoming a successful adult. Teachers often strengthen this idea, doing everything they can, as they teach the knowledge and skills required to be successful, to teach children to look at life more seriously.

Children do need to learn that there's more to life than play, and that there is a time to play and a time to be serious. But I am convinced that we go too far when we demand so much from kids that they lose their ability to be playful. We produce adults who have are unable to lighten up—even when it's appropriate. In my humor seminars and workshops, I ask the audience to get up and do some playful and silly things (mooing like a cow, talking as if they have a ping pong ball in their mouth, etc.). There are generally some people who stiffen up and glare at me for putting them in such an embarrassing situation. Others are very comfortable and just go with the flow and have fun with any silly activity thrown their way.

Which camp do you fall into? Are you easily embarrassed when you do something at odds with your image of yourself as professional, competent, serious, and respectable? If so, then you'll want to spend extra time on the Second Habit. If not, you're probably already comfortable being playful. But you should still complete the Humor Log exercises designed to nurture the Second Habit to further strengthen the "elf" within yourself.

When you become more playful, you also become more spontaneous and get more enjoyment from what you're doing at the moment. And in this frame of mind, things just naturally strike you as being funnier than they do when you're more serious.

> **A woman at a singles dance keeps sneezing, and can't seem to stop. A guy walks up to her and asks if she's OK. She says, "Yeah, I've been sneezing for five minutes."**
>
> **"God, that's terrible!" says the guy. And she sighs, "Well, it's not that bad, because each time I sneeze, I have an orgasm."**
>
> **So he says, "Wow! Are you taking anything for it?" "Yeah," she says, "pepper!"**

Your goal should not be to become someone who's always playful and never serious. This isn't very adaptive, and is one of the things your parents and teachers worked so hard to overcome. If you are generally very serious, your initial goal should be to recapture the ability to be playful in just a few situations. Once you have achieved that, you can focus on learning to shift from a serious to a playful style of interaction whenever you choose, or whenever the situation calls for it. You want to become more flexible in this sense—able to easily switch gears and create a playful mood.

The Meaning of a Playful Attitude

What does it mean to have a playful attitude? Many adults are clearly not playful when they're playing. We use the term "play" to refer to such activities as tag, football, soccer, cards, chess, playing the piano, etc. By the time you enter school, play becomes competitive and goal-oriented, and you're anything but playful. You're determined to win, or at least do well, when playing. This is not the kind of play that forms the core of your sense of humor.

The dictionary defines play as any activity that is amusing, fun, or otherwise enjoyable in its own right; i.e., it is intrinsically enjoyable. There is no particular goal you're trying to achieve. Once the focus shifts to an outcome (pleasing someone, doing better than others, achieving a specific level of performance, etc.), it stops being fun. It may even become work!

> *"You are led through your lifetime by the inner learning creature, the playful spiritual being that is your real self."* (Richard Bach)

Since much of the stress in your life comes from the hassles and minor problems that are there every day, you're never really free from stress. Learning to be more playful, even in difficult situations, will help you lift yourself out of the stress of the moment, leaving you in a better position to roll with the punches life throws your way.

Begin thinking of a playful attitude as a skill, as well as a habit. The key idea here is getting yourself to the point where you are able to take control over when you are and are not playful, rather than having it hinge on whether good or bad things are happening in your life, or whether you are around positive or negative people.

Why is a Playful Attitude the Foundation for Your Sense of Humor?

We all inherit a basic biological disposition toward playfulness, and this shows up in different ways as we move through childhood and adolescence, reflecting the development of new intellectual and social skills. [For a detailed discussion of the development of children's humor, see my book *Understanding and Promoting the Development of Children's Humor.* For a description of this book, see www.LaughterRemedy.com.]

A boy came home with a report card that included four D's and three F's. He said, "What do think my problem is dad, heredity or environment?"

Humor is most likely to be experienced when you're mentally playful. That is why the Second Habit is so important in improving your sense of humor. As you become more comfortable with (and skilled at) being playful, your natural sense of humor (re)emerges.

"When you're depressed, the whole body is depressed, and it translates to the cellular level. The first objective is to get your energy up, and you can do it through play. It's one of the most powerful ways of breaking up hopelessness and bringing energy into the situation." (O. Carl Simonton, M.D.)

Some people, however, lacking this playfulness, never learn to lighten up; they enter their senior years in an expanding web of bitterness, anger, anxiety, or depression at the unfair path life has given them. Others simply have a vague sense of regret or longing; a sense that they've somehow missed something important by being so serious all their life. This is demonstrated by an 85-year-old woman in the hills of Kentucky, who said:

"If I had my life to live over, I'd make more mistakes this time. I'd relax; I'd limber up. I'd be sillier than I've been this trip. I'd take fewer things seriously . . . You see, I'm one of those people who live sensibly, day after day . . . If I had it to do over again, I'd travel lighter than I have."

This woman clearly regrets the lack of playfulness in her life, but feels it's too late to change. If you recognize yourself in her, don't wait until you're 85 to realize that the quality of life improves when you become more playful. This book will help you avoid her fate.

I know of one woman who described herself as pretty serious most of her life; but her sense of humor blossomed as she got older (she lived to be 98). She was a very religious person, so she was always aware of how much she had to be thankful for. "After all," she said, "Just think of where I'd be if wrinkles hurt." George Burns, who died at the age of 100, once said, "You can't help getting older, but you can help getting old." Who better demonstrates the power of humor to prevent "hardening of the attitudes?"

Using Props to Induce a Playful Attitude

If you've been a serious person most of your life, you'll need all the help you can get in strengthening the Second Habit. Silly toys and props will help you out. Make it a point to go out and buy several. They can be anything that brings out your sense of fun, silliness, or playfulness. One woman I know keeps a set of wind-up false teeth in her desk. When wound up, the teeth just sit on her desk going "clackety-clackety-clackety-clack." She says it always helps her lighten up when things get tough.

A corporate Vice President who I taught to juggle scarves says that when the tension gets too high on her job, she closes her door, gets out the scarves and spends a few minutes juggling. She becomes totally focused on the scarves and quickly gets caught up in the fun of it. It has helped her lighten up every time she's tried it. Maybe blowing bubbles will work for you, or a silly hat, or cartoons, or a silly buzzer. Silly noses work well for me, partly because of the reaction I generally get from other people when wearing them (I have 30 different animal noses).

"The supreme accomplishment is to blur the line between work and play." (Arthur Toynbee)

If you have a management position, try keeping a few silly props sitting on your desk, file cabinets, book case shelves, etc. People who've done this find that when employees come in, either to complain or just to talk, they generally go over and unconsciously pick up a toy or prop and start fiddling with it. You can see their tension ease as they play with it. For most of us, such brief playful respites elevate our mood and leave us in a better frame of mind for effectively doing our job.

Humor Log: Things to Do and Think About

Record your responses to the following in your Humor Log.

On Play and a Playful Attitude

1) What does it mean to be a playful person, or to adopt a playful attitude in life?
2) Does it make sense to distinguish between playful and serious forms of play? How do they differ?
3) How will learning to become a more playful person help develop your sense of humor?
4) Plato once said, "Life should be lived as play." How would you interpret this?
5) Think of people you know who are serious all the time. Write down as many words as you can which describe these people.
6) Think of people you know who have a playful attitude, but are still competent and professional in their work. Write down as many words as you can which describe these people. Compare the qualities you listed here to those listed in 7).
7) What negative views of playful adults do many people have?
8) A well-known saying states, "We do not stop playing because we grow old; we grow old because we stop playing." How can a loss of a playful outlook on life make us grow older?
9) It's important to learn when a playful response is not appropriate. List a few examples of such situations.
10) Describe the benefits you would receive from becoming a more playful person.

Work and Play

1) Describe the dichotomy between work and play in our culture. Are these really incompatible with each other? Can a playful attitude actually help you be more effective on the job?
2) Do you have fun at work? What would it take to make your job fun? Answer both in terms of changes in yourself and changes in the work environment.
3) How is a lighter attitude on the job viewed where you work?
4) Discuss the notion of seriousness in connection with competence, professionalism, and responsibility. Do these three qualities require that you always be serious on the job?

5) How does Terminal Seriousness set you up for greater stress on the job and in life generally?
6) Discuss the difference between taking your work seriously and taking yourself seriously.
7) Would increased opportunities for humor and fun on your job make you more or less productive? Why?

Current Playfulness

1) How often are you playful in everyday life?
2) When you are playful, who are you generally with, and what are the circumstances?
3) When you are serious, who are you generally with, and what are the circumstances?
4) What makes you uncomfortable about being playful (if that's true)?
5) All things considered, what do you expect your biggest obstacle to be in adopting a more playful attitude toward life?

Early Development and Influences

1) How playful/serious were you as a child? As an adolescent?
2) When did you lose the playfulness of your childhood?
3) Were there any early events that caused you to become a less playful person than you would like to be? Focus specifically on parents and teachers, along with other pertinent life experiences.

Group Session

Opening Fun Activity

Have a game or fun activity prepared to put the group in a playful mood. Consider having a "twit race," as shown on the old *Monty Python* television programs. Or assume that the Minister of Silly Walks has come to your meeting and requested that everyone walk across the room with their best silly walk. Assign someone to be prepared for an opening activity for the next meeting.

Discussion of Home Play for the First Habit

The Home Play for the First Habit should be discussed before moving on to a discussion of the Second Habit. Sample discussion ideas are listed below. (Consult your Humor Diary to jog your memory about key insights while working on the First Habit.)

1) Share with a partner the ways in which you immersed yourself in humor during the past week(s).
2) What new insights have you had about your sense of humor, as a result of doing the Home Play for First Habit?
3) Now that you've spent a week or two thinking about your sense of humor, have your goals in going through the Seven Humor Habits Program changed?
4) You can also use the beginning of this session to discuss any topics from the First Habit that you didn't get to last time.

Discussion of the Second Habit

Use the general material presented in this chapter, including items from the Humor Log exercises, to generate a discussion of play and a playful outlook on life. Be sure to also talk about the general importance of a playful attitude for improving your sense of humor. Remember to stay in touch with your telephone partners.

Home Play

1) Do the Humor Log exercises.
2) Take a silly photo of yourself. Keep it with you or put it in a place where you'll see it every day. Use it as a reminder to maintain a playful attitude.
3) Make a list of things you have fun doing and do two each day. Don't restrict it to big things like skiing, scuba diving, or traveling in Europe. Also include little things, like walking in the park, going to movies, playing backgammon, and having a drink with friends.
4) Spend time watching young children play. If you have forgotten how to be playful, think back to what you were like as a child. If you have young children of your own, be more attentive to how they play. Pay special attention to their spontaneity, joy, and absorption in the moment.
5) Put reminders to be playful in key places (bathroom mirror, refrigerator, office, car, etc.).
6) Find a prop (silly nose, toy, etc) that gets you in a playful mood. As you use your props, notice how they help pull you out of a serious or somber mood and create a lighter, more positive mood.
7) Whenever possible, hang around positive people. In a *Peanuts* cartoon, Linus asks Lucy, "How did you like Disneyland?" Lucy coolly answers, "I didn't. They didn't have marmalade for my toast." It's difficult to be playful when you're around negative, complaining, irritable people all the time.
8) Make it a point every day to do something playful that is out of character for you. Face the rear of the elevator while everyone else is facing the front, wear a funny prop, ask someone at random for their autograph, pay a toll for the person in the car behind you, etc. Be creative, but avoid tasteless pranks.
9) Catch other people in the act of being playful. Be on the lookout for playfulness in other adults. Keep a tab of the number of examples you spot each day.
10) Be sensitive to where a playful attitude is and is not appropriate. And be sure to continue taking your work and responsibilities seriously while cultivating playfulness.

THE THIRD HABIT

LAUGH MORE OFTEN AND MORE HEARTILY

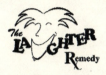

"What soap is to the body, laughter is to the soul."

(Yiddish proverb)

ZEN BUDDHISTS BELIEVE THAT IF you start the day off with a laugh, you'll be fine the rest of the day. These days, hundreds of laughter clubs around the world get together regularly for 10 or 15 minutes of laughter exercises, following the "laugher club" tradition started in the 1990s by the Indian physician, Dr. Madan Kataria. The twenty years I spent as a researcher studying humor and laughter led me to respect the wisdom of this view. Even if you're laughing when there's nothing to laugh at, this generates the playful frame of mind where humor lives; and the laughter itself may well offer some direct health benefits.

When you lighten up and have free access to joyful laughter, you become more resilient—more stress resistant. In fact, I think of *laughter as a "stress deodorant."* With the rising stress levels in most people's lives these days, you're going to need repeated applications of this deodorant every day.

Laughter certainly has an energizing effect, helping you fight burnout and lethargy at the end of the day. And most people say they just feel better—sometimes even euphoric—after a good laugh. (We now know that part of this good feeling results from the fact that humor and laughter activate known pleasure centers in the brain.)

Learning to laugh more often and more heartily, then, is essential to taking full advantage of the stress-reducing (and resilience-inducing) power of humor.

A staff member at a hospital told me following one of my seminars that she was once asked while under hypnosis to start laughing and to just keep on laughing. She did this for several minutes. When brought out of the hypnotic state, she reported having "the best feeling I've ever had in my life." She said she felt totally relaxed, but also "energized and up." You'll find the same effect occurring within you even when you're not hypnotized.

"The unexamined life is not worth living." (Socrates)

"Life without laughter is not worth examining." (Paul McGhee)

Research has demonstrated that going through the motions of the behavior associated with a particular emotion actually causes you to begin to experience that emotion. That is, by acting as if you're angry or happy, you actually begin to feel angrier or happier. Even making the facial expression that generally accompanies an emotion increases the extent to which that emotion is felt—especially happiness.[1] Laughter has the power to pull your emotions in a more positive direction, even when you're exposed to something that would normally make you angry or anxious.[2] It helps you take control of your emotional state, and that very control reduces stress.

An 80-year-old woman said her cancer had been in remission for over 30 years.
I asked her what she attributed her long life to. She said, "Well, I haven't died."

Life is like an elevator. Some days you go up, some days you go down, and some days you get the shaft.

These findings support the familiar advice to "Let a smile be your umbrella," or "Put on a happy face." Your emotional memories are connected to physical movements, so the movements themselves revive part of the experience of past similar emotions. They may not be as strong, but if you have a strong emotion that's close to the surface, going through such actions can bring it back vividly. To get a sense of how this works, do exercise #3 under "Belly laughter" in the "Group Session" at the end of this chapter.

"Time spend laughing is time spent with the gods." (Japanese saying)

If you are not much of a laugher, you should make the effort here to laugh more heartily when you do find something funny. The easiest way to practice this is in situations where your own laughter gets lost in the laughter of a crowd (e.g., at a party or movie). Make it a point to notice how you feel after a good laugh in these situations. Non-laughers often say that this helps them become more expressive in general—both with positive and negative emotions.

"Laughter lets me relax. It's the equivalent of taking a deep breath, letting it out and saying, 'This too will pass.'" (Odette Pollar)

If you have a CD player in your car, you have an ideal means of practicing laughing every day. By listening to comedy CDs on the way to and from work, you can regularly strengthen the habit of laughing, making a natural and hearty laugh more and more accessible. This will help you ease into laughing more freely in social situations.

"There are three things which are real: God, human folly, and laughter. The first two are beyond our comprehension. So we must do what we can with the third." (John F. Kennedy)

As you work on belly laughter for the next week or two, keep an eye out for the "anti-laughter police." Every organization has them. These are people who know that if you laugh on the job, you can't possibly be working or taking your job seriously. You'll recognize them from the hostile glances thrown your way when you are caught laughing. Use their reactions as a reminder that you work in a setting where laughter is not always viewed positively. At the same time, remember that they may be right. Learning to judge when laughter is and is not inappropriate is an essential humor skill to develop. So be sure to choose the right time and place to work on the Third Habit.

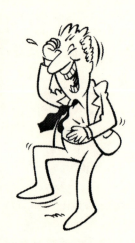

Humor Log: Things to Do and Think About

Again, record your answers in your Humor Log.

1) When you have a good belly laugh, how does it make you feel? Before you answer this, get a partner and do nonstop belly laughter for 20–30 seconds (do whatever is necessary to keep yourselves laughing). Then pay attention to any physical or other changes you notice.

2) Name three people you know who you consider "good laughers." Compare their personalities to others who laugh less often or less heartily.

3) Have you ever had the experience of laughter suddenly turning into crying? Why does this sudden reversal of emotions occur? How do you feel after such a laugh/cry?

4) Many consider laughter on the job inappropriate in any situation. Describe areas of your job or work setting where laughter would be inappropriate, even if you did find something funny. Under what circumstances would laughter be acceptable?

5) Assume that you have a job that requires you to be on the phone a lot. Your boss (amazingly enough) has suggested that you have a brief laugh as you lean over to pick up the phone (but stop before you answer it). What effect might this have on how you're perceived by the caller?

6) Describe how you think laughter helps reduce stress.

Current Laughter

1) How often do you have a real belly laugh?
2) Describe your typical laughter (quiet, explosive, etc.).
3) On a typical day, how many times do you laugh out loud?
4) How emotionally expressive are you in general? Is your laughter "style" consistent with this? Do you think learning to have a good belly laugh more often can help you become more emotionally expressive in general? Why or why not?
5) What would you like to gain during this week or two, in terms of how often you laugh, and how heartily you laugh?

Early Development and Influences

1) During your childhood and adolescence, did you laugh a lot? (Ask your parents, or an aunt or uncle, if you don't remember.)
2) Describe your mother's and father's laughter, both in terms of how often and how heartily they laughed.
3) What influence do you think the laughter patterns shown by your parents had on your own laughter?

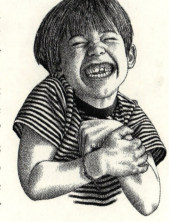

4) Describe your parents' general emotional expressiveness and how that might have influenced your emotional expressiveness.
5) Did your parents ever get upset at your laughter (e.g., because you were laughing too much, or too loudly)? How often? Did they sometimes ask you to just stop laughing so much? How did this influence the development of your own laughter style?

Group Session

Opening Fun Activity

Discussion of Home Play for the Second Habit

Consult your Humor Diary for reminders about your insights or observations while working on the Second Habit.

1) Open with a request for a show of hands of those who contacted their telephone partner during the week to discuss the Home Play. Remember that regular contact with your partner boosts the benefits received from this Program, since it helps keep you actively engaged.

2) Share with a partner your list of "fun things to do." Which of these activities were most effective in boosting your playfulness?

3) What progress did you make toward becoming more playful? What new insights did you have regarding your playfulness?

4) Discuss your observations of young children playing. What qualities did they show in their play that you lack?

5) What props or reminders did you use to help establish the habit of adopting a playful outlook in life? Bring one to show to the group.

6) How did your friends, family, and colleagues react to your efforts to become a more playful person?

A Laughter Imagery Exercise

Use any of the material discussed in connection with this Habit, along with the Humor Log exercises, to generate issues for group discussion. Also try the following exercise (to be led by one group member). Leave as much time between suggestions as seems appropriate. Introduce any other variations that make sense to you.

"Close your eyes . . . Let a big smile slowly grow on your face . . . Now let your face go back to its usual expression . . . Now go back to the smile . . . Go back and forth between these two expressions. Notice any changes in how you feel . . . Now clench your jaw and fists . . . Notice how that feels . . .

Keep your jaw and fists clenched, and start breathing quick, short breaths . . . Notice how that feels . . . Now think back to a time when you had a good long belly laugh. It could be a very recent time, or a time from your childhood . . . Picture the situation as vividly as you can . . . What other people are there? . . . What happened that got you started laughing? . . . Let out a little giggle when it feels right to do so . . . Let the giggle build up, and gradually lead into belly laughter . . . Now think back to a particular time when you were really depressed . . . Hold your body in the way you usually do when you're depressed . . . Say 'I'm depressed' to yourself (and mean it) . . . Turn to the person on your right and left and say, 'I'm so depressed.'. . . Hang your head down . . . Hunch your shoulders over . . . Keep your arms close to your body . . . Stand up right at your chair . . . Take a few depressed shuffling steps, without leaving your chair . . . Now start exaggerating your depressed behavior . . . Let your shoulders drop lower than anyone would ever do . . . Make your depression really extreme . . . Now start adding some silliness to your depression . . . Be playful as you act depressed . . . Now forget about being depressed, and just start being silly in any way that suits you . . . And that's a good place for us to stop."

After completing this exercise, discuss the impact of making yourself engage in such behaviors as smiling, tightening your jaw and fists, laughing, acting depressed, and exaggerating depression in a playful way. What emotions did these actions make you feel (if any)? Can you influence how you feel by simply getting yourself to behave in a way associated with one emotion or another? What implications does this have for the value of forcing yourself to smile or laugh more than you usually do?

Home Play

1) Do the Humor Log exercises for the Third Habit.

2) Laugh more often and more intensely than you usually do.

3) Seek out social situations (e.g., at movies and parties) where you will have the opportunity to practice belly laughter without feeling conspicuous.

4) Get a few comedy CDs and practice laughing when alone in your car. Force it if you have to. This will gradually make it easier to belly-laugh spontaneously and naturally.

5) Put up reminders (where you're sure to see them) to laugh more than you usually do when an opportunity arises. Leave them up until laughing starts to seem more natural and spontaneous.

6) Use silly props to help keep you in a frame of mind which is naturally conducive to laughter.

7) Spend more time with people who make you laugh.

8) Tell friends, family members, and colleagues at work that you will be making an effort to laugh more than you usually do. Also tell them why, and ask for their support.

9) At some point, try forcing yourself to laugh (get a friend to join in with you) when you're angry, anxious, or depressed. Notice the effect this has on your emotional state.

10) Continue thinking about situations where your laughter comes easiest and where you have to force it a bit. Remember to jot down ideas and observations related to the Home Play in your Humor Diary.

The Fourth Habit

Create Your Own Verbal Humor

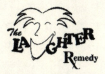

"Wit is the sudden marriage of ideas which, before their marriage, were not perceived to have any relationship."

(Mark Twain)

PLAYWRIGHT GEORGE BERNARD SHAW ONCE wrote to Winston Churchill:

"Dear Mr. Churchill,
    Enclosed are two tickets to my new play, which opens Thursday night. Please come and bring a friend, if you have one."

Churchill sent back the following reply:

"Dear Mr. Shaw,
    I am sorry, I have a previous engagement and cannot attend your opening. However, I will come to the second performance, if there is one."

As a child growing up in the 1950s, I loved to watch Groucho Marx on his television show, *You Bet Your Life*. One day he was interviewing a woman from Iowa, and she said she had eight children. Groucho said, "Eight kids. That's amazing. How come you have so many kids?" The woman answered, "Well, I guess my husband just likes me." Without hesitation, Groucho quipped, "I like my cigar too, but sometimes I take it out!" (Groucho, known for pushing the limits with his humor, lost his TV show because of this spontaneous comment.)

Churchill, Shaw, and Groucho were known for their quick wit. You're probably not yet ready for this level of spontaneous wit, but if you have immersed yourself in humor during the past few weeks, and are now both more playful and a better laugher than you used to be, then you are ready to take the first step toward creating your own humor. Many people want to skip the first three steps, because they seem to have little direct bearing on humor skills. But in the long run, you'll make faster and more lasting progress if you take the First, Second and Third Humor Habits "seriously." They give you the basic foundation you need to be successful in the Fourth Habit—especially if you haven't used humor much in your life.

Learning to create your own verbal humor will be of tremendous value in using your sense of humor to cope with life stress. The basic strategy adopted here is to ease into the habit of creating your own puns and other simpler forms of verbal humor by first telling memorized jokes—and doing so on your good days, when you're not under stress. Once you develop the habits of effectively delivering memorized humor, and then spontaneously playing with the meanings of words on our own on your good days, the ability to make up your own verbal humor gradually will start showing up under more stressful situations.

Ignoramus: Someone who doesn't know something you've just learned.

"What's the difference between ignorance and apathy?"
"I don't know and I don't care."

Most people going through the 7HH Program should choose to *split their work on these two aspects of verbal humor, spending a week or two on each one.* They go together very naturally, though, so the first will naturally easy into the second. If you're already a great joke teller, then you can spend less time with this—or skip it completely.

Begin Telling Jokes and Funny Stories

You may have long ago given up on being able to tell a joke or funny story well. Perhaps you've tried in the past, only to find people looking at you blankly. So you decided that some people just don't know how to tell jokes—and you're one of them!

"A joke is not a thing, but a process, a trick you play on the listener's mind. You start him off toward a plausible goal, and then by a sudden twist, you land him nowhere at all or just where he didn't expect to go." (Max Eastman)

Or maybe you've just never made the effort. In that case, you'll be pleasantly surprised at how easily you can weave jokes into conversations without really appearing to tell a joke—once you've made the effort to memorize jokes and practice telling them. For example, if you're in the midst of a conversation about the harmful effects of smoking, you can directly ease into lines like this: "A smoker I know has read so much about the harmful effects of smoking that he decided to give up reading."

A Jewish doctor who removed foreskins dies, and his wife discovers a bag of 100 of them in a drawer. His daughter takes them, saying, "I know a guy who makes things, maybe he can do something with them." So she gives them to this guy and comes back a couple of weeks later to see what he's done with them. He shows her a wallet. "A wallet?" she says, "100 foreskins, and that's it?" "Ah, but if you rub it, it becomes a suitcase."

Art Buchwald once said, "I learned quickly that when I made others laugh, they liked me. This lesson I will never forget." Everybody likes people who make them laugh, but becoming a good joke teller will do more than make you popular and entertaining. It will also improve your communication skills and help you manage conflict more effectively, both within your family and at work. A former assistant secretary general of the United Nations noted that jokes are even used in diplomatic negotiations and receptions to ease tensions.[1] Henry Kissinger, President Nixon's secretary of state in the 1970s, frequently used jokes to break through the icy tensions surrounding negotiations with the Soviets during the cold war. (I know, for those of you who remember him, it's hard to imagine Kissinger telling jokes; but if he can do it, you can do it.)

"I don't make jokes. I just watch the government and report the facts."
(Will Rogers)

In 1987, a tremendous amount of tension surrounded the upcoming SALT talks with Gorbachev and the Soviet Union. As the meetings began, Reagan told the following joke to Gorbachev:

Moscow is having a lot of problems with people driving too fast. So the city police have been issued strict orders to give a ticket to anyone caught speeding. One day Gorbachev is late getting to the Kremlin, so when his driver comes to pick him up, Gorbachev says, "You sit in the back, and let me drive. We'll get there faster."

So they take off. Pretty soon, they zoom past a couple of motorcycle cops. One of them speeds out after the car. A few minutes later, he comes back, and his partner asks, "Well, did you give him a ticket?"

He answers, "No, I didn't."

"What?" says the partner, "Why not? Who in the world was it?"

"I don't know, but his driver was Gorbachev!"

Gorbachev loved the joke, and it immediately began to break down the barriers between the two men, helping establish a climate conducive to more effective negotiations. It will work the same way for you as you negotiate your life.

If you've never tried to tell jokes in the past, start with one joke—and be sure you think it's funny! The first thing to do is memorize it. How many times have you heard people start to tell a joke, only to forget the punch line? This is the most common mistake made by novice joke-tellers. One way or another, they butcher the punch line. If this sounds like you, begin by telling the joke to a few close friends, your spouse, or anyone else with whom you feel totally comfortable. This will minimize your embarrassment, in case you do mess it up. Remember, good friends include anyone who—when you make a fool out of yourself—feels you haven't done a permanent job.

"If you want someone to laugh at your jokes, tell him he has a good sense of humor." (Herbert V. Prochnow)

After practicing with your friends, begin telling the joke to work associates (when the circumstances are appropriate, of course). A good way to create opportunities to practice your jokes is to simply ask people if they've heard any good jokes lately. Those who like jokes will welcome the opportunity to tell a few. And after they've told one, you'll have a natural opportunity to tell one yourself. This also gives you a chance to learn some new jokes.

If someone else tells a joke that you think is especially funny, write it down at that moment. Keep a small notebook in your pocket for just such occasions. If you don't write it down, you'll forget it. Or you may remember part of it but not know it well enough to repeat to someone else. Consider putting the joke on a 3" x 5" index card (so you can carry it around in your pocket for a while) or in your computer when you get a chance. If you use a spread sheet on your computer, you can even organize the jokes by content or any other dimension you choose. Develop a collection of jokes you like. This will keep you focused on building up your joke repertoire.

When I heard the following joke, I didn't hesitate. I immediately grabbed a piece of paper and scribbled it down.

A couple that had been married 55 years was watching a faith healer on TV. The evangelist said, "I can heal you tonight brothers and sisters! I can heal you

tonight! If you want to be healed, put one hand on the television and the other on what you want to heal."

So the woman put one hand on the TV and the other on her tired old heart and prayed along with him.

The man looked over and thought to himself, "Well, what have I got to lose?" So he put one hand on the TV and snuck the other between his legs.

His wife looked over at him and said, "He said he could heal, not raise the dead."

If you lead meetings or are a teacher, you may want to remember certain jokes because they demonstrate a point that you know you'll want to make from time to time. You'll be amazed at the impact the joke has when it's directly linked to the topic you're discussing at the moment. I loved the just-mentioned joke, and (sometimes) use it in talks to senior citizens when I want to lead into stereotypes about sexuality among the elderly or concerns about aging.

If you have no way of writing the joke down, make it your top priority to remember the punch line. This is the most crucial part of the joke. You'll be able to reconstruct the joke well enough later to make it funny—even if it's not exactly the way you heard it.

When you get to the point where you feel comfortable telling one joke, simply add another. Adding only one or two jokes at a time to your repertoire, and practicing them a lot before learning new ones, will assure that you won't forget the old ones as you add new ones. Be sure you're comfortable with the first jokes before adding others. Being relaxed and confident about joke telling is an essential part of being a good joke teller.

"Act as if you enjoy telling the joke, which suggests you know how to do it." (Leo Rosten)

You can make many jokes funnier by changing some of the details so they're more salient to the person or group you're telling them to. Will Rogers, the early 20th century American humorist, once said, "I'm not a member of an organized political party . . . I'm a _____." You could say either "Republican" or "Democrat," depending on who you're talking to. If you are going to poke fun at a group, however, make sure the person or group you're talking to is not a member of it, or doesn't identify positively with it. Otherwise, the joke will not only fall flat, you'll also offend your audience.

Everyone knows someone who just can't tell a joke. The following classic joke pokes fun at these people.

> **A new convict is sitting in his cell at the state prison. Suddenly, someone yells out, "42!" The whole cell block starts laughing. Someone else yells, "125!" Again, everyone laughs. "74!" Mass hysteria. This goes on all afternoon, and the new guy can't figure it out. He asks his cell mate what's so funny.**
>
> **He says, "We've been telling the same jokes so long that everybody knows all the jokes. So we just gave them numbers, and call out the numbers."**
>
> **So the new guy thought he'd get into the act, and called out, "82!" But nothing happened. Total silence. He tried again, "77!" Again, no reaction. He asked his cell mate why nobody laughed. "Well," his partner answered, "Some people just don't know how to tell a joke."**

In the late 1980s movie *Punch Line*, an aspiring comedian (played by Tom Hanks) has consistent success on stage until some "significant" people come to check him out for a possible shot at the big time. He uses material that has always worked for him in the past, but nothing works for him on the one evening that it's essential that he get good laughs. Everything he does is flat. The reason? The pressure caused him to loose his spontaneity and playfulness. He's not relaxed and natural. The more desperate he gets to produce something that's funny, the worse it gets.

You may experience a form of performance anxiety yourself if you're new at telling jokes. That's why you want to start with a single joke or two, and tell it over and over among friends until you feel totally comfortable with it, and know how people are generally going to react. This experience among friends will strengthen your ability to keep a naturally playful demeanor in delivering the joke to strangers, as well.

You may want to choose a few jokes told by your favorite comedians, and imitate their style and delivery. Just as artists copy the masters before they develop their own style, you can copy good joke tellers' style before developing your own.

While working on jokes, try your hand at stories, as well. The following is one of my favorites.

> **During World War II, a British pilot is shot down and captured by the Germans. He has serious injuries from the crash, and the Germans say, "We're going to have to amputate your right leg." The pilot says, "OK, if you've got to do it. But do me a favor. Could you just drop the leg along with your bombs the next time you bomb London? At least part of me would be home." They say, "Ya, we can do that for you."**
>
> **A week later, it's the same story with his left leg. Again, he asks the Germans to drop the leg over London on their next bombing mission, and they say, "Ya, we can do that for you."**
>
> **A couple of weeks later, they tell him they're going to have to amputate his right arm, and he again asks if they can drop his arm over London. To his surprise, this time the Germans say "Nein, this we cannot do." So he asks, "Why not? You were willing to drop each leg over London."**
>
> **They say, "The Gestapo thinks you're trying to escape!"**

In collecting and memorizing stories, always ask yourself, "What point can I make using this story?" For example, in this case, you could use the story to illustrate how absurd our reasoning can become when we get caught up in our own limited view of things. A line of reasoning that makes sense in some situations can be complete nonsense in others.

When personalizing jokes, be sure that the changes you make

don't destroy the humor. Otherwise, you'll be in the position of the Englishman who decides that he wants to learn a typical American joke to take back home, because he thinks Americans have a great sense of humor. Somebody gives him the following (simple) joke:

"What does a fat man do after he runs for a bus? He takes off his hat and pants."

When he gets back to England, he says, "I heard this terrific joke in America. What does a stout fellow do after he runs for a tram? He takes off his cap and trousers."

One of the most important rules in the list on the next page is to always keep in mind when humor is and is not appropriate. Failure to be sensitive to the social situation can put you in the position of the politician who would always walk over and start telling stories whenever he saw a little group of people gathered together. After capturing people with his story, he'd make his political pitch. It worked pretty well most of the time, but one day he ran into a group that just wouldn't warm up to him. He said, "What's the matter with you folks? You act like you were at a funeral." A member of the group looked up at him and said, "Brother, this is a funeral."

"Forgive, O Lord, my little jokes on Thee, and I'll forgive Thy great big one on me." (Robert Frost)

41

General Rules for Communicating Humor

If you have no experience at telling jokes and stories, use the following guidelines to maximize your chances of success.

1) Don't try to tell jokes/stories that you don't know well.
2) Don't tell a joke you don't find funny yourself.
3) Don't laugh at your own joke (especially in advance).
4) Don't announce, "This is a joke," or "I'm not very good at telling jokes, but . . ."
5) Don't apologize if others don't laugh.
6) Don't try to explain the joke if people don't laugh. It still won't be funny.
7) Use gestures and facial expressions while telling the joke.
8) But don't feel obliged to act funny while telling the joke.
9) Be clear about which words need emphasis.
10) Don't drag it out! Remember, brevity is the soul of wit.
11) Be sure the punch line is at the end. Don't telegraph what's coming.
12) When the joke invites visualization, pause to allow your audience to imagine the situation.
13) Don't overdo puns. They're generally less funny to the hearer than to the teller.
14) Keep your humor positive.
15) Avoid sensitive topics and put-down or other potentially offensive humor—especially among people you don't know. Remember that others' sensitivities may differ from your own. You may offend people and not know it.
16) Avoid racial and sexist humor.
17) Know your audience before attempting "risky" humor.
18) Be sensitive to the social situation; know when any humor at all, or a particular joke/story, would be in bad taste.
19) Know when to stop joking and be serious. Nothing is more frustrating than trying to communicate with someone who refuses to take you seriously.
20) Personalize or localize jokes when possible. Use names, activities and locations familiar to your audience.

Humor Log: Things to Do and Think About

Record your answers in your Humor Log.

On Joke and Story Telling

1) What do you think are the most important qualities distinguish a good from a poor joke/story teller?
2) Why is it so difficult for some people to remember jokes and stories? What can you do to help yourself remember them?
3) How important do you think joke telling is, in comparison to skills associated with the other habits in this program? Why?

Current Joke/Story Telling

1) How often do you tell jokes or funny stories on a typical day? Would you like to do so more often?
2) How would you describe your skills as a joke or story teller? If you're not good at it, what generally goes wrong?
3) How would you like to improve your joke-telling skills?

Early Development and Influences

1) How often did you tell jokes or funny stories during your a) childhood and b) adolescence? Again, ask your parents about their memory of this. (If your parents are no longer living, ask anyone else who was around you a lot as you were growing up.)
2) Do you now tell jokes more often or less often than you did as a child/adolescent? When/why did this change occur?
3) How often did your mother and father tell jokes or funny stories when you were growing up? What impact did this have on you?
4) How do you recall your parents reacting to the riddles and jokes you told as a child? Did they generally react positively or negatively? Were they supportive of your early efforts at humor? Did this have any effect on the development of your joke-telling skills or habits?

Puns: The Foundation for Your Verbal Sense of Humor

We all grew up enjoying puns. In my generation, the puns from childhood took the form of moron (a term now agreed to be insensitive and unacceptable) jokes and knock-knock jokes. The following will be forever etched in my memory.

Why did the moron bury his car? The motor was dead.

Why did the moron tiptoe past the medicine cabinet? He didn't want to wake up the sleeping pills.

Why did the moron jump off the Empire State Building? He wanted to try out his new spring suit.

What is black and white and red (read) all over? A newspaper. (You should be able to think of other answers.)

Knock knock. Who's there? Gorilla. Gorilla who? Gorilla (girl of) my dreams, I love you.

Knock knock. Who's there? Arthur. Arthur who? Arthur any stars in the sky tonight?

We've all heard the phrase, "The pun is the lowest form of wit." So why use puns as the starting point for learning to create your own verbal humor? Because this is where you probably left off in developing your sense of humor during childhood or adolescence. Children first begin to understand puns around the age of six or seven and go through a period of several years tirelessly telling riddles based on puns. Interest in riddles then fades because they just aren't as funny as they used to be. They're too simple!

Types of Puns

Several kinds of word play can be classified as puns.

1) Same spelling, same pronunciation.

In some puns, the key word is spelled and pronounced the same way for both meanings.

Working in the garment district is a seamy business.

What did Samson die of? Fallen arches.

2) Different spelling, same pronunciation.

When ordered to row the lifeboat, the first-class passenger harrumphed, "Do I have a choice?" "You certainly do," replied the sailor, "either oar."

To be successful, a doctor has to have a lot of patience.

Every time the prince found a girl he thought might be Cinderella, he went down to defeat. (This is not a pure case.)

3) Different spelling, different pronunciation.

Note that each of the key words in these examples are themselves real words.

Death is just around the coroner.

Male jogger to female jogger: "My pace or yours?"

Someone who always tells the same joke has a one-crack mind.

The Eskimos are God's frozen people.

Oliver Wendel Holmes once said that he was grateful for small fevers.

"Hanging is too good for a man who makes puns; he should be drawn and quoted." (Fred Allen)

Yet we all know a chronic punster who hits us with one pun after another. And what is the predictable reaction? A groan! While there are exceptions, most puns just aren't very funny to adults, precisely because they're so simple. It's no coincidence that the word "pun" forms the first half of the word "punish." And that's exactly what you're doing to your listener when you overuse puns. Tell anyone you catch overdoing puns that if they do one more, you'll see that they do time in a "punitentiary."

The reason persistent punsters never get the message that their puns aren't very funny is that they really are funnier to the person who creates them than they are to those who hear them. It's more difficult to have the quick insight that leads to creating a spontaneous a pun than it is to understand it when someone gives it to you on a silver platter. People who are always thinking of puns tend to be impressed with how clever they are—and they really are more clever than the rest of us, at least in this sense. But that doesn't change the fact that their puns generally aren't very funny.

"In the beginning was the pun." (Samuel Beckett)

So we're left in the paradoxical position of puns being funniest to the person who produces them. As Oscar Levant once put it, *"A pun is the lowest form of humor—when you don't think of it first."* Why, then, should you spend a lot of time developing this skill if no one's going to appreciate it? Because your ability to play with words will serve you well when you're under stress. It will become a powerful tool in helping you manage your mood every day. It will help you take control over your emotional state, instead of leaving it to the mercy of the good or bad things happening to you on any given day. Remember, the purpose of this program is to help you learn to use your sense of humor to cope with difficult life situations, not to entertain other people with your finely-honed wit—although this also will occur as you move through the program.

Think back to when you were a child. How often did you make up your own puns? If you were like most kids, the answer is "rarely, if ever." [My book, Stumble Bees and Pelephones, helps kids build their skills at creating their own riddles based on puns. It will also help you get started with this step if English is not your native language. See www.LaughterRemedy.com to order.] You just kept repeating the jokes and riddles you heard. When you did make up your own, they bombed. Instead of laughter, you got strange looks. Or, if you told them to adults, you got a good laugh because they made no sense at all. This is why special attention is given to puns here. Puns are basic foundation-level verbal humor skills.

How to Develop Your Ability to Create Verbal Humor

There are several things you can do to improve your ability to come up with your own spontaneous puns and other verbal humor. If you practice the exercises included here and in the Humor Log exercises section at the end of the chapter, playing with language soon will become second nature to you.

An Exercise in Multiple Meanings

People who are good at creating their own spontaneous humor are very quick at seeing other possible meanings of a key word or phrase during conversations. The rest of us know these other meanings but don't have the habit of simultaneously seeing both meanings, because the context always makes the intended meaning clear. If you've never been a playful thinker, *your starting point should be to focus your attention on extra meanings of a word as soon as it's spoken.*

A good way to heighten the quickness of your thinking along these lines is to take words associated with common objects or events and try to think of two or more ways of interpreting them. This does not produce jokes, but strengthens your ability to see and create extra meanings. And a greater awareness of multiple meanings will enable you to create your own spontaneous jokes. Think of this as a preliminary habit that will strengthen your verbal humor habit in the weeks ahead.

The next page provides a few examples. To practice this exercise, look at objects in the room you're now in and try to come up with words which have two or more possible meanings. Also try to imagine verbs which lend themselves easily to double meanings. Write down

Chair	• Something you sit on • A position or title (e.g., chair of a committee)
Table	• A piece of furniture • To table a motion • Water level
Pen	• A writing implement • A place to keep pigs • A female swan
Book	• A written document • A record of bets • A set of cards • Engage someone's services
Fan	• Something used to keep you cool • Someone who follows sports • To spread something out • To strike out (baseball)

To accelerate your progress, make a game out of this. Practice the exercise while driving, waiting for the bus, walking down the street, etc. This has far more value than you would guess. It strengthens the habit of having surplus meanings quickly pop into mind. You may have to force yourself to do the exercise at first, but you'll quickly reap the rewards.

Look for Word Play on Public Signs

Humor is often used on public signs to capture attention. For example, a sign in a funeral parlor said, "Ask about our layaway plan." A jewelry story in a mall had a sign out front saying, "Ears pierced while you wait." A furniture store displayed a sign saying, "Modular sofas—only $299. For rest or foreplay."

The signs listed below were found in a broad range of business establishments. To practice your skill at thinking in terms of puns, first cover the right column and try to guess what kind of business would be associated with each sign in the left column. Then look at the right column. The businesses in this column are listed in the incorrect order. (The answers are listed below.)

Sign	**Location**
1. **Ask about our layaway plan.**	A) Plumber's truck
2. **Get lots for little.**	B) Hair stylist
3. **Come in and have a fit.**	C) Funeral parlor
4. **Curl up and dye.**	D) Lumberyard
5. **Medium prices.**	E) Restaurant
6. **Better laid than ever.**	F) Fortune teller
7. **Litany candles?**	G) Real estate office
8. **A flush is better than a full house.**	H) Catholic church
9. **If you're at death's door, let our doctors pull you through.**	I) Toilets
10. **Don't stand outside and be miserable. Come in and get fed up.**	J) Poultry farm
11. **Come see, come saw.**	K) Hospital
12. **#1 in the #2 business**	L) Shoe store

Answers: 1C, 2G, 3L, 4B, 5F, 6J, 7H, 8A or L, 9K, 10E, 11D, 12I.

Look for Ambiguity in Everyday Conversations

Make a conscious effort to find ambiguity in conversations—both your own and those of others. Don't worry about whether it's funny or whether it's intended as a joke. Just look for words where a second interpretation is possible. The context of most ambiguous statements makes the intended meaning clear. But humorists trick us by using the other meaning—even if it appears to make no sense at all.

You never know when you'll accidentally say something which could be interpreted in another way. I once did a program for a group in a church basement, and had just finished talking about looking for ambiguity in conversations. I noticed a small organ over in one corner of the room during the break and innocently said to the minister (who was participating in the workshop), "Gee, what a beautiful little organ you've got." Five women standing nearby cracked up, immediately practicing what I had been preaching.

Most of the time, the extra meanings you notice won't be very funny. Don't worry about it; that's not the goal here. You're taking the initial steps needed to put the detection and creation of puns on automatic pilot. If you spend a week or so devoting some time every day to listening actively for ambiguity, you'll quickly get better at spotting double meanings, even when you're not looking for them. They'll just jump out at you. For example, a friend of mine heard this announcement from a pilot just after takeoff from Chicago: "We'll be cruising at 37,000 feet and briefly pass out over the lake." She thought the remark was very funny, but noticed that no other passengers seemed to have spotted the unintended meaning.

A doctor was asking a woman questions in an attempt to find clues about the cause of her persistent abdominal pain. He asked, "Are you sexually active?" She answered, "No, I just lay there." The doctor controlled his laughter, but was laughing on the inside. Another doctor told a 16-year-old that she had acute vaginitis. She looked down with embarrassment and said, "Thank you."

"There is a foolish corner in the brain of the wisest man."

(Aristotle)

Since you are not used to seeing ambiguity in language, it will take an active effort to get into the habit of doing so. To speed up the process, use the same notebook you used to copy down jokes you like. Every time you hear or see a word (on signs, in conversation, in a newspaper, etc.) containing ambiguity, write it down, along with enough of the context to enable you to remember it later. This will strengthen the habit of noticing ambiguous communications, even if you never tell them to anyone else.

A few examples are given below to give you the basic idea. Take the underlined word, or set of words, and substitute another word, or set of words, which has basically the same meaning. But the word(s) you substitute should produce an ambiguity in the meaning of the sentence. For example, you could take the phrase, "He went lion hunting with a group of friends," and change it to, "He went lion hunting with a club." The second sentence is ambiguous, while the first one is not. *Avoid looking at the ambiguous versions (which follow immediately after the set of unambiguous versions) until you've tried to create your own ambiguous way of restating the sentence.*

Unambiguous Sentences

1) She helped the boy <u>put on</u> the hat.
2) He laughed <u>in</u> school.
3) He saw a <u>ferocious</u> shark.
4) The <u>sailor's heavy wife</u> likes to cook.
5) The duck <u>can now be eaten</u>.
6) The mayor asked the police to <u>not allow</u> drinking while driving.

Ambiguous Versions

1) She helped the boy with the hat.
2) He laughed at school.
3) He saw a man-eating shark.
4) The heavy sailor's wife likes to cook.
5) The duck is ready to eat.
6) The mayor asked the police to stop drinking while driving.

Look for Humor in Newspaper Headlines

Most American newspapers have adopted the habit of inserting word play into some of their headlines. If your newspaper does this, developing the habit of looking for double meanings in headlines will further strengthen your own sensitivity to ambiguity.

The following exercise (using the technique developed for my book, *Small Medium at Large*) involves real headlines taken from newspapers. A key word or two has been left out of each headline. Your task is to fill in the blank with a word that makes the headline funny. Make the effort to come up with your own answer before checking the answers given below. Use the clue given only if you need it. Remember, your answer could be different from the one given here, but be just as funny. You'll know you're making progress when the humor in such headlines begins to automatically pop out at you in reading your own newspaper. As you become familiar with the pattern of word play used here, try coming up with your own headlines. You can use this skill to build some fun into office memos, announcements of meetings, etc.

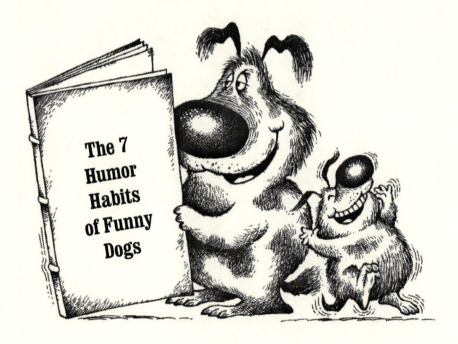

The 7
Humor
Habits
of Funny
Dogs

Puns

1) **"Condom week starts out with a _____."**
Clue: It's a good start. The word is also slang for a verb meaning "to have sex."

2) **"Man shoots alligator ____ pajamas."**
Clue: This is a little word, but still makes it funny.

3) **"Organ recital fades after _____ beginning."**
Clue: An excellent or solid beginning.

4) **"Pants man to expand at the _____."**
Clue: A men's clothing store is enlarging the present store—not at the front, but . . .

5) **"'Family _____ fire just in time,' chief says."**
Clue: They find or spot the fire.

6) **"Trees can _____ wind."**
Clue: Weaken or reduce. Think of a childish prank that's always in bad taste (actually, another sensory system is closer).

7) **"Drought _____ coyotes to watermelons."**
Clue: Causes them to start eating watermelons.

8) **"Ban on nude dancing ____ Governor's desk."**
Clue: This is another little word, but it does carry the pun.

Absurdity

9) **"Furniture drive for _____ launched."**
Clue: What group of people does it make sense to raise money for, but not furniture?

10) **"Man _____, _____; death by natural causes ruled."**
Clue: A cause of death that is anything but natural.

Stating the Obvious

11) **"Researchers call _____ a threat to public health."**
Clue: The most extreme assault on one's body possible.

12) **"'Death row inmates no longer allowed day off after _____,' official says."**
Clue: The one condition in which a day off is irrelevant.

13) **"Commissioner says _____ is needed to end drought."**
Clue: What's always needed in a drought?

14) **"Women's Club to hold June meeting in _____."**
Clue: None needed.

Answers to Newspaper Headlines

1) Bang	8) On
2) In	9) Homeless
3) Firm	10) Shot, stabbed
4) Rear	11) Murder
5) Catches	12) Execution
6) Break	13) Rain
7) Turns	14) June

Daffynitions

In daffynitions, the idea is to use some aspect of a word to come up with a really daffy definition of the word. Daffynitions are an admittedly low level of humor, but learning to generate them on your own is an excellent way to build your ability to see ambiguity and play with language. Again, you can do this any time you're in a situation where you have a few minutes with nothing to do (waiting in line, riding a bus, waiting for your meal in a restaurant, etc.). Just look around the room for ideas for different verbs and nouns, and find as many as you can which are conducive to daffynitions. You can use newspapers, magazines, or any other printed matter as a source of words to play with.

A dictionary is the best starting point for this exercise. Go through the pages at random looking for words which seem ideal for daffynitions. I picked up the dictionary while writing this and opened it up at random to "O." Here's what he came up with:

Oar: What you are when you borrow something.
Oblate: When you don't go to sleep until the wee hours.
Oboe: When you've borrowed someone's bow.
Ode: Made a long time ago.
Odor: A person who sings odes.
Offense: Where something that used to be on the fence is when it falls.
Ooze: What people say when they see a beautiful sunset.
Oppose: What you do when you go to a photographer.
Orchid: A kid who likes to row boats.
Oregon: Row the boat one more time.

I purposefully wrote down the first thing that came into mind as I thought of these words. With more reflection, I could probably have come up with funnier lines. Other answers are also possible. The point is that, if you do the same thing and just verbalize the first daffynition that you think of, you'll get better at having this kind of word play occur to you automatically. Create your own daffynitions of the following (see below for some possible answers):

- Alarms   • Arrears   • Crock   • Delight   • Fungi
- Insane   • Mutilate   • Vitamin   • Debate   • Zebra

Practice Generating Your Own Punch Lines

The best way to learn to generate your own puns and other jokes may be to practice creating your own punch lines in already-created jokes. The examples on the next page are given to help you see how you will benefit from practice at creating your own punch lines. Fill in the blank with any word or phrase that creates ambiguity within the context of the other information given. There often is more than one acceptable answer, so if yours differs from the one given, do not consider it wrong. Also, don't worry about how funny your answer is. If it creates ambiguity, that's all that matters at this point. (All of these examples were taken from my book, *Small Medium at Large*, also published by AuthorHouse. That book provides several hundred opportunities to practice this skill.)

Answers to Daffynitions

- Alarms: What an octopus is.
- Arrears: What we often forget to wash behind.
- Crock: A Japanese device for telling time.
- Delight: What you turn on to see in da room.
- Funghi: A guy who knows how to have a good time.
- Insane: Where Parisians swim on hot days.
- Mutilate: What tomcats do at night.
- Vitamin: What you do when guests visit.
- Debate: What you put on de hook.
- Zebra: The biggest bra they make.

---

1. **(A classic) "Waiter, what's this fly doing in my soup?"**
   "I don't know sir, but it looks like _____."
   Clue: Look for a second meaning of "doing."
2. **What would it take to legalize marijuana these days?**
   A _____ session of congress.
   Clue: What are marijuana cigarettes called?
3. **A couple of women walk into a club for men only, and the waiter says, "I'm sorry ladies, we only serve men here."**
   One woman replies, "_____."
   Clue: Look for a second meaning of "serve."
4. **Did you hear about the two angels who got kicked out of heaven? They were trying to _____ a _____.**
   Clue: This is a double pun. A familiar phrase meaning to "earn a profit."
5. **What does a grape say when you step on it? Nothing, it just gives a little _____.**
   Clue: You probably don't need one. In case you do, think of a term for an unpleasant way young children cry.
6. **How are a duck and an icicle alike? They both grow ___.**
   Clue: What duck product is used in ski jackets?
7. **"The Police Department reported today that someone broke into police headquarters during the night and damaged their toilet facilities**. The sabotage remains a mystery, and at present the police have nothing to _____."
   Clue: None needed.
8. **There is a new potency pill for men that works better than Viagra, but it has one drawback. If it's swallowed too slowly, the user winds up with a _____ neck.**
   Clue: A slang term used to refer to a dead person.

Answers to Generating Your Own Punch Line

1) The backstroke

2) Joint

3) Good, we'll take two

4) Make a prophet

5) Wine

6) Down

7) Go on

8) Stiff

Exaggeration

Exaggeration is another technique that will serve you well under stress. If you exaggerate your problem to extremes—to the point that it becomes ridiculous—it's easier to find a way to laugh at it. And this helps you let go of the problem instead of carrying it around. Therapists know the value of exaggeration. Every year, more therapists are learning to use it to help patients cope. Alan Fay points out in his book, *Making Things Better by Making Them Worse*, that therapists sometimes use exaggeration to pull patients out of depression. (See Appendix 1 for a discussion of research showing the effectiveness of the 7HH Program in reducing depression.)

One woman was very depressed about her husband's heart attack and death. She felt responsible, because she had been pressuring him to do work around the house when he got home. A logical approach by the therapist failed to take away her guilt. She kept saying, "If only I had treated him better . . ."

One day, after a remark like this, her therapist said, "That's right. We have to face the fact that you killed him. It was clearly murder. The only decent thing to do is turn yourself in at the nearest police station." She chuckled and improved quickly after this.

If you're prone to being anxious in the midst of everyday problems and hassles, try exaggerating the way you usually react. For example, shake your hands, breathe rapidly, pace back and forth, shouting something like, "Oh my God! Oh my God! This is it! This is the end! I'm dead. I'll never get out of this!" For extra effect, say it in a high-pitched, or otherwise silly, voice.

"Comedy has to be truth. You take the truth and put a little curlicue at the end." (Sid Caesar)

Exaggeration is commonly used by comedians. Johnny Carson, a popular late-night American talk show host for about 30 years (replaced years ago by Jay Leno), was famous for his "It was so hot/cold/small/large that . . ." lines. Here are some examples.

Exaggeration Jokes

I had a cavity so deep that my dentist sent me to a podiatrist. (A Woody Allen joke)

My ranch is so big that when I go for the mail I have to pack a lunch (take a change of clothes, etc.).

It was so hot that when the dogs chased cats, they both walked.

He's so old, the bank mails him a new calendar one month at a time.

Sampson was so popular, he brought down the house. (Notice how this exaggeration joke differs from the others.)

He's so clumsy, he trips over cell phones.

I had so many zits when I was a kid, the blind always wanted to read my face.

He was so rich, he bought his dog a boy.

Michael Iapoce, in his book *A Funny Thing Happened on the Way to the Board Room*, describes the following excellent 5-step technique for learning to create your own exaggeration jokes.

1) Pick a subject. It could be yourself, your mother-in-law, school, your job, marriage, your car, anything at all. Let's say you pick your car.

2) Make a list of associations to this subject, using only nouns. For "car," you might come up with door, headlights, engine, trunk, windshield wipers, gas tank, license plate, speedometer, wheels, dash, chrome, paint, hood, glove box, tow truck, etc.

3) Pick an adjective to describe the subject. It might be old, slow, small, economical, etc. Let's pick "old."

4 Make another list of associations for the word selected in step 3. These generally should be nouns, but some verbs also will work. For old, you could include wrinkles, Geritol, fossils, antiques, Roman numerals, grey hair, arthritis, stone carvings, hieroglyphics, Dead Sea Scrolls, liver spots, petrified wood, prunes, bifocals, false teeth, etc.

5) Find words within the two lists that you can meaningfully connect. Connect them in a statement that makes sense in an exaggerated or absurd way. Practice this exercise by using one of the terms listed in step 4 to complete the following sentences. Cover up the right column below now, and try to come up with your own answer (sometimes more than one answer works).

Exaggeration Exercise

My car is so old that the:

1) Headlights . . .	have bifocals.
2) Gas tank . . .	uses prunes.
3) Speedometer . . .	is in Roman numerals.
4) Paint . . .	has wrinkles.
5) Engine . . .	runs on Geritol.
6) Chrome . . .	has liver spots.
7) Dash . . .	is petrified wood.
8) License plate . . .	is carved in stone.
9) Trunk . . .	contains dinosaur eggs.

Now repeat the exercise on your own in your Humor Log. To maximize the benefit, repeat it several times. (Note: this is much more fun when done with another person.)

Humor Log: Things to Do and Think About

Record your answers in your Humor Log.

On Play with Language

1) Why do we generally groan at puns?
2) When do children start to understand puns?
3) Are all riddles and puns alike? How would you classify them?
4) Why do puns generally seem funnier to the person who creates them than to the person s/he tells them to?
5) Can learning to create your own puns help sensitize you to spotting other forms of humor in everyday life? How?
6) How will learning to play with language help you cope with stress?
7) If you were to become more skilled at creating humor, how might that improve your job performance?
8) List a few situations where you've seen coworkers make witty remarks that were inappropriate. Why were they inappropriate?

Current Verbal Sense of Humor

1) Do you enjoy puns and other forms of word play? Why (not)?
2) How often do you produce original puns in conversations?
3) What is the most common form of verbal humor you initiate?
4) Do you prefer to make up your own spontaneous verbal humor or tell memorized jokes and stories?
5) How often do you create your own verbal humor at work? What keeps you from doing this more often on the job?
6) How important is it for you to improve your skill at creating puns and other verbal humor?

Early Development and Influences

1) Did you go through a period between 1st–3rd grades during which you constantly told riddles? If possible, ask your parents, or anyone else who knew you as a child. What prompted you to tell fewer riddles and jokes as you got older?

2) Was there any other period in your childhood or adolescence during which you told a lot of jokes?

3) As you look back at your life (including your adult years), at what age were you most prone to creating your own spontaneous verbal humor? Why do you think you did more then than you do now?

4) When you told jokes while growing up, were they generally memorized, or did you often create your own spontaneous jokes?

5) When you did initiate some form of humor as a child or adolescent, what kind of humor was it generally?

6) Who had the greatest (positive or negative) influence on your ability to create verbal humor?

7) How did your mother and father influence your ability to create humor?

Group Session: Joke Telling

[Since there is so much material on verbal humor, it is suggested that groups spend separate sessions on jokes/stories and spontaneously-created verbal humor. Accordingly, separate Group Session and Home Play sections are provided here.]

Opening Fun Activity

Open the meeting by asking each person to tell their favorite joke.

Discussion of Home Play for the Third Humor Habit

What were your experiences in your efforts to laugh more often and more heartily? How did you go about it? Did you force laughter at first? Did this forced laughter help you "break through" so you could laugh more openly and heartily? Did it seem unnatural? Did laughter gradually become easier and more comfortable? What situations did you use to practice laughter? What reminders did you use? Consult your Humor Diary for ideas for discussion.

Telling Jokes

1) Use jokes told at the beginning of this session as a basis for discussing what is and is not funny (to you). Also give the people who told jokes feedback on how well they told them. What could they improve in terms of delivery of the joke?
2) Ask for volunteers to tell jokes in ways that assure that the joke won't be very funny. Then discuss what was wrong with the delivery.

Home Play: Joke Telling

1) Learn and tell one new joke each day. Be sure you think it's funny. Rehearse it. Be sure you have it memorized before telling it to someone else. Tell it to as many people as you can.

2) Ask your friends and people you work with to tell you their favorite joke or funny story. Develop the habit of asking them periodically if they've heard any good jokes lately. People welcome the opportunity to tell jokes, and it opens the door for you to practice telling your own jokes. Be on the lookout for jokes you find especially funny. When you hear a joke you want to remember, do either of two things:

A) Keep your Humor Diary with you, and immediately (or as soon as possible) write it down. You can even ask the person to repeat it so you can get it written down.

B) If the joke is not long, and you can easily remember it, tell it to someone else at the first opportunity. This will help solidify it in your memory. Once you've told it three or four times, you'll have it.

3) Listen to CDs or watch DVDs of your favorite comedians. Select a few of their jokes that you think are funny, and practice telling them to your friends. Imitate their delivery style.

4) Continue to focus on being more playful than you have been in the recent past. Make it a point to be in a playful mood when practicing your joke-telling.

5) Continue being playful and laughing more than you usually do.

6) Record your joke-telling observations in your Humor Diary.

A doctor's wife is unable to sleep because the toilet is dripping. So she has her husband call the plumber. The plumber listens, but then grumpily declares, "But its 2 a.m.!" And the doctor says, "So what? If your child were sick, wouldn't you call me? "You're right," says the plumber, "so I'll tell you what to do. Throw a couple of aspirins in the bowl, and if it's not better in the morning, call me."

Group Session:
Spontaneous Verbal Humor

Opening Fun Activity

As in the last session open the meeting by asking each person to tell a new joke (one learned since the last session) that they find very funny. If a group member shows more confidence and skill in telling the new joke than was shown in telling a joke in the previous session, be sure to provide positive feedback to that person.

Discussion of Home Play for Joke Telling

Discuss your successes and failures at learning, remembering, and telling jokes since the last session. How did you decide which jokes you did and did not want to remember? When you were not successful, what seemed to go wrong? Did you restrict yourself to learning just one new joke a day or try to learn several at one time? As the group describes their own experiences in learning and telling jokes, look for common problems that several group members seemed to have and discuss these.

Did you write new jokes down in your Diary when you heard them, or rely on your memory alone? Did any friends offer you feedback on what you did wrong in telling some of your jokes? If so, share this feedback with the group. Have each group member indicate the number of jokes s/he now feels comfortable telling at a moment's notice.

Did you listen to CDs of professional comedians since your last meeting? If so, which ones? Did you practice imitating their delivery? Did this seem helpful in discovering your own joke-telling "style?"

Finally, discuss whether you were able to keep a light and playful style in telling jokes. This generally works best but you may also discover that you are more comfortable with a more serious "tongue in cheek" approach.

Creating Your Own Verbal Humor

Be prepared to talk about any of the issues raised in the Humor Log exercises for the Fourth Habit. Also practice or discuss any of the exercises presented above during the session. Come prepared with your own variations of these exercises. Give special consideration to the following:

1) The exercise in "multiple meanings" provides a good starting point. Break into smaller groups of four or five people. Take turns giving a target word. One person names a common word, of which s/he can think of at least two meanings. The person to his/her left then gives one meaning, the next person gives a second, etc., until no one can think of any more meanings. Remember that although these are not jokes, it helps stimulate the habit of quickly thinking of alternative meanings. The exercise moves more quickly if someone brings a prepared list of words with multiple meanings.

2) If you want to play a version of "daffynition," make it a point to have a dictionary available at this session (to make it easier to co me up with words conducive to good daffynitions). Play the game in groups of 8-10 people. Group members will take turns saying a word for which they have a daffynition in mind. The rest of the group then says out loud whatever daffynition they think of. As soon as no more ideas come forth, the next person proposes a new word to be given a daffynition. Doing this in a group will help you get started creating them on your own.

3) Do the "Cartoon Caption" exercise, described above.

4) Try the five-part technique for creating your own exaggeration jokes, described above.

HOME PLAY:
SPONTANEOUS VERBAL HUMOR

1) Complete as many of the exercises included in this chapter as you can. The more effort you put into it, the more rapidly your verbal humor skills will develop. A lot of exercises have been included for this habit specifically to give you ample opportunities to practice this key skill. Spend as much time as necessary to give yourself the feeling that you've made real progress on this Fourth Humor Habit before going on to the fifth.

2) Do the "Exercise in multiple meanings" at least once each day. Do it when you're in your car, waiting in lines, eating alone, riding the bus, etc. Writing the meanings down is not essential. But be sure to probe your mental dictionary for extra meanings. Even if you only have a few minutes, you'll benefit from this exercise.

3) Look for ambiguous words or phrases in conversations. Put reminders to do this in places where you'll see them. Whenever possible, write them down (this will help strengthen the habit of looking for them) in the same pocket-size notebook you used to record jokes. Include enough of the context to enable you to fully remember them later. At the end of the day, consult your notebook and think about the ambiguities you noticed that day. Ask yourself which ones were funny and which weren't.

4) Also record any examples of word play you notice in

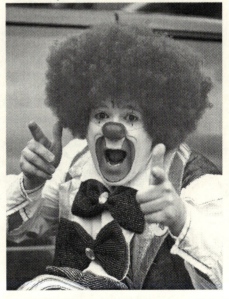

Why do cannibals refuse to eat clowns? Because they taste funny.

newspaper headlines and on signs. Jot these down in your notebook.

5) Spend one day out of the week creating daffynitions. Do this whenever you have a few spare moments (at lunch, lunch, waiting in the doctor's office, in elevators, etc.). Jot your daffynitions down in your notebook. Make a game out of it by engaging others in it.

6) Be on the lookout for communications in which you can take what is said literally and produce a comic effect. For example, if someone told you to "keep your eye on the ball . . ." Also keep looking for funny literal interpretations of headlines (e.g., "Drought turns coyotes to watermelons.").

7) Generate as many spontaneous puns as you can during conversations. Start with family members or friends (anyone with whom you feel comfortable taking a risk). Don't worry about how funny they are. Just get into the habit of playing with words.

8) Find some time to work on the "Exaggeration exercise" described in this chapter. Since this exercise is a little more difficult, do it with a friend in order to make it fun.

9) Get a book of captioned cartoons and create your own captions. Be sure to cover the existing caption first, or you'll find yourself unable to think beyond the caption given. Do this with a friend or two, if possible. Get into the habit of looking at the cartoons in your daily paper, and of creating your own caption for at least one of the cartoons every day.

10) Stay in touch with your telephone partners.

11) Be sure to use your Humor Diary to keep track of your own efforts at creating verbal humor, including what worked and did not work (in terms of getting others to laugh).

THE FIFTH HABIT

LOOK FOR HUMOR IN EVERYDAY LIFE

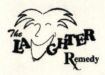

"You can't really be strong until you see a funny side to things."
(Ken Kesey)

ONE OF THE MOST EFFECTIVE ways to get the health benefits of humor, and to eventually learn to use humor to cope with stress, is to improve your skill at finding a funny side of things that happen in everyday life. If you have done the Home Play for the first four habits, you should already be better at doing this. Becoming more playful puts you into a frame of mind that makes it easier to see the funny side of things. Even when you are being serious, it's probably much easier now to switch gears and become playful than it was before you started the 7 Humor Habits Program. And while you may not realize it yet, joke telling and looking for word play in everyday conversations, newspapers, and on signs, also helps you get started seeing the funny side of situations that have nothing to do with language.

The goal of the Fifth Habit is to sensitize you to the opportunities for humor on your job, at home, in the grocery store, in your relationships, and in every other facet of your life. You will learn to spot humor where you least expect it. A few years ago, I was watching a PBS television program on "Madness" and the history of psychiatric approaches to treating it. The announcer read: "Madness is made possible by the Corporation for Public Broadcasting and viewers like you." I howled with laughter, and scrambled to write it down before it was forgotten.

You are exposed to such opportunities for humor every day, but you're simply not seeing them. Some years ago, the first time I noticed a pay phone on a plane, I remember being seized with a mid-flight urge to call Dominos Pizza and have a pizza delivered. A flight attendant told me that a man once complained to her about the design of the lavatories on the plane. He said that some turbulence had occurred while he was urinating, and he didn't have anything to hang on to. She had to restrain herself from saying, "Well, blame Mother Nature, it's not our fault."

You soon will have thoughts like this popping into your own mind, as you work on the Fifth Habit. But you will have to spend a couple of weeks—maybe a month—making an active effort to find humor everywhere you go before you begin to notice it without trying. Developing this habit when you're not under stress is one of the most important things you can do to prepare yourself to find humor when you are under stress.

I heard this same flight attendant walk down the aisle with a cup of decaffeinated coffee asking, "Who asked for the unleaded?" Most of the people within ear shot of her flashed a big smile. It was a brief comment, made in passing while carrying out her regular duties. It took no extra time, but added just a little bit of happiness to the lives of the passengers. It's these seemingly minor everyday opportunities for humor that are the most important to work on.

"All eyes are on Mrs. Kennedy as she picks her seat."
(Radio commentator's words about Jacqueline Kennedy, wife of President John F. Kennedy, at a public event in the 1960s.)

I was listening to the radio recently and reference was made to former President Reagan's Memoirs, which were published in the 1990s. I remembered that he was known for his memory lapses during his presidency, and I laughed out loud as I had a completely different take on the notion of his memoirs. My laughter, stopped, however, when I also recalled that he developed Alzheimer's disease in his later years.

It's easy to find ready-made humor these days. The internet provides an endless source of jokes and funny stories on almost any topic or incident. And, of course, there are sit coms and comedy films on television, funny TV ads, stand-up comics on TV and in clubs, regularly appearing cartoons in newspapers and magazines, funny newspaper columnists, etc. But while the packaged humor that is thrown at you daily does help ease stress, it's not the most effective way to manage stress through humor. It comes at the end of the day, and not when you're in the situations that cause stress (at least job-related stress). And it has no meaningful connection to those situations. Also, it's passively received humor, rather than actively produced . . . by you!

To use humor to cope, you need to take a more active role in creating or finding your own humor. The problem is that you may still be at ground zero when it comes to finding humor in your own life. You never see it because your head is full of more important things—like what you're going to have for lunch, when the coffee machine will get fixed, and the fact that you drive your son's friend more often than his parents drive your son when the two of them have to go somewhere.

"From there to here and here to there, funny things are everywhere."
(Dr. Seuss)

Be sure to start looking for the light side of non-stressful situations before doing so in stressful ones (doing this while stressed out will come later). This includes simply spotting life's oddities when they occur. For example, Charlie Chaplin once entered a Charlie Chaplin look-alike contest, and came in third. A New York City couple was mugged and had their money, jewelry, some clothes, and a pair of tickets to a Yankee baseball game stolen. They reported the theft to the police. On a hunch, the couple went with the police to the game that the tickets were for. Incredibly, the muggers were sitting in their seats—and one was wearing the husband's cool leather jacket! Who could fail to see the humor in this?

Five or six railroad cars filled with chlorine derailed a few years ago, posing a threat to the surrounding community. A string of barriers was set up to prevent anyone from getting near the restricted zone. No one was allowed near because of the danger. But then the Governor showed up, and the on-site coordinator gave him a close-up tour of the scene. I immediately thought of the way canaries used to be taken into mines.

I once spotted a newspaper article about a company in Colorado called "Dog-Gone." This enterprising company developed a vacuum system for sucking prairie dogs out of their holes and into a large tank on a truck. "The animals are deposited alive 'but somewhat confused' into the tank". The mere image of a giant vacuum cleaner sucking prairie dogs out of their holes makes me chuckle.

Looking for humor will take extra time and mental effort at first. But after a week or two of putting "finding humor" on the front burner, you'll discover that it takes less and less time and effort. Soon, it will take no extra time at all. You'll notice things that make you laugh while remaining fully engaged in the activity of the moment. That's when humor really begins to serve you and becomes a tool for dealing with stress. At that point, humor gives you back the energy that stress-induced anger, anxiety, and depression steal from you. The more you immerse yourself in the Fifth Habit, the more quickly you will see this change in yourself.

What is a Humorous Perspective?

We all have different mental perspectives on the world. Men and women, teenagers and adults, Republicans and Democrats, etc., all have different perspectives on life because they bring a different set of ideas or starting points for viewing and making sense of things.

Mental perspective also is important in another way. Look around the room you're in right now and find five things that are round. Now find five things that are red. These things were there all along, but you didn't see them—because you weren't looking for them. You didn't have a mind-set to see "round" or "red."

The same thing happens with humor. You are surrounded by situations all day long where you might find something funny—if you have a mind-set to look for it. In working on the Fifth Habit, you will learn to do the humor-equivalent of asking yourself, "What are the round things in the room?"

"What did the Zen Buddhist say to the hot dog vendor?"
"Make me one with everything."
When he received no change for his $5 bill, he said, "What about my change?"
"Ah," said the hot dog vendor, "change must come from within."

So what does it mean to have a humorous perspective on life? How does the head bone get connected to the funny bone? How do humorists think that's different from the way you think? First, they have the ability to quickly switch from a serious frame of mind to a playful one. This makes it easy for them to see a light side of things that others miss. Second, they have more unusual associations to events, and are more willing than the rest of us to turn the world upside down for the fun of it. They enjoy toying with crazy ideas. This helps sustain a high level of mental flexibility and creativity.

"An egg is funny. An orange is not." (Fred Allen)

People with a well-developed humorous vantage point on life enjoy creating absurdities in their own minds. Sid Caesar was one of my favorite comedians during my childhood in the 1950s. He could take a common innocuous situation and make it absurd. In a skit on the old *Show of Shows*, he took his child to the movies on a cold winter day and put so many clothes on him that you could hardly see the child. When they got back home, he took off the child's hat, ear muffs, mittens, coat, another coat, boots, leggings, sweater, a second sweater . . . When he finished, there was no child there.

In another skit, he played a woman putting on her make-up. He draws a line on the right eyebrow, and then the left. After scrutinizing them, he decides the right one is too short, so he lengthens it. Then the other one is too short, so he lengthens it. This continues to the

73

point where he finally has lines coming all the way down the sides of his cheeks. And the audience is howling.

Humorists also have a built-in tendency to see and enjoy the incongruities, ironies, absurdities, and ridiculous aspects of real life. They thrive on the oddities of things that happen and that people do, like the following:

> **A bank robber in a small town was caught recently after signing his name to a withdrawal slip just prior to the holdup.**

> **A man in Texas had been hiding from the law for 17 years. He finally got caught when he contacted the FBI to find out if they were still looking for him.**

> **After his surgery for gallstones, a man awakened in his hospital room to discover the stones on the same tray on which his medications had been placed. A nurse had put them there so he could see the cause of his torture. With some effort (thinking they were medicine), he finally got them down.**

Learning to spot these events yourself is one of the most important skills you can develop. If it helps, try assuming that God has a great sense of humor, and that He has set up opportunities for you to laugh every day. Your job is to enjoy the chances He gives you.

Getting Started

How do you get yourself to the point where you notice the funny side of things if you're not used to doing it? There are several easy things you can do.

Put up "What's Funny about This?" Reminders

If you rarely find humor in your life, the best way to begin is by doing something that helps you remember to look for it. Put up reminders in key places (refrigerator, desk, car, etc.) to actively look for funny things in situations where you don't normally see any.

Focus on daily routines and circumstances. At the beginning, you'll have to be very specific and ask, "Is there anything weird, incongruous, surprising, ironic or absurd about this?" Or you may be more comfortable simply asking yourself, "OK, if I were (name your own favorite comedian), what would I find funny about this?" With practice you won't have to consciously ask yourself. You automatically will notice the light side of things that happen.

Have a chuckle at the things children say out of naiveté. A friend of mine heard her daughter say, "there's today, tomorrow, and tonow." You might also hear gems like these:

> **A little boy and girl were getting a bath at the same time. The girl says, "Can I touch it?" The boy answers, "No, 'cause you broke yours off."**

> **A mother trying to save money on the bus (children have to pay if they're over five) hurries her daughter past the driver, but he says, "Just a minute little girl, how old are you?" "Four and a half," says the girl. "And when will you be five?" "Just as soon as I get off this bus."**

A hospital I spoke at in New Jersey had a separate division of the hospital on Madison Avenue, in another part of the city. A shuttle bus carried employees back and forth between the main hospital and the Madison Avenue building. Painted in large letters on the side of the vans were the words, "MAD Employees Shuttle."

Make it a point to ask yourself, "What's funny here?" even for mundane occurrences. If you can't find anything funny, change the question to, "How could I change this situation so that it would be funny?" Feel free to exaggerate or distort circumstances, including what people are doing and saying, so that it does become funny.

Ask Friends/Colleagues about the Humor They See

Some of your friends or colleagues may already have a well-developed sense of humor and may be very good at noticing the funny side of things. Seek these people out while working on the Fifth Habit, and spend more time with them than you normally do. Whenever you see them, make it a point to ask about the funny things they've noticed recently. Talk to co-workers about the humorous things they've noticed. People who enjoy humor usually enjoy sharing it, and the funny things they notice will help sensitize you to seeing humor in the same things yourself.

A hospital employee told me recently that someone had posted on a bulletin board an article which said that "Research shows that the first five minutes of life are very risky." Someone had penciled in below it, "The last five minutes aren't so hot either." She also said that the intensive care unit of the hospital is often referred to as either the "intensive scare" or "expensive care" unit.

"If you smoke, don't exhale." (Sign observed in a taxi)

Someone else told me about a couple of horses named "We're Not Sure" and "Who You Gonna Call?" entered in the same race. Amazingly enough, they finished first and second. The announcer called out, "As they come to the wire, it's Who You Gonna Call and We're Not Sure!"

Write it Down

Whenever you notice anything that strikes you as funny, write it down at the first opportunity. Use any scrap of paper you can find, and then record it later in your Humor Diary. If you don't have time to get the details down at the moment, write a key word or phrase as a reminder to record it in detail later. This will help keep you from forgetting it.

One of the most innovative uses of humor I've seen came up in a junior high school basketball game. The evening sports news showed highlights of a game that was tied with about three seconds to go. One of the teams had the ball out of bounds under its own basket. Just before the ball was thrown in, a player on the in-bounding team got down on his hands and knees and started barking like a dog. The other team was momentarily distracted, and a teammate took the pass right under the basket and made an easy shot to win the game. It was hilariously funny and creative. I wrote it down immediately.

"I think I have old-timers disease."
(Remark by an elderly patient, overheard in a hospital.)

The reason for writing things down is not to share them with others later (although this is a good idea, as noted next), but to reinforce the habit of noticing humor.

Share the Humor You Observe

Sharing the funny things you see is another powerful way to build up the habit of noticing humor. If you're new at this, make sure it's something you feel most comfortable with—for whatever reason. Also make sure you found it funny yourself. Mention it to everyone you come in contact with. By telling the same story over and over again, you'll rapidly improve your ability to make it interesting as you tell it. As soon as you feel like you've mastered that one, start with another one and repeat the same procedure.

"I see humor as food . . . An adequate share of humor and laughter represents an essential part of the diet of the healthy person."
(Norman Cousins)

When doing this, remember that some funny things that you see just won't be as funny when you describe them to someone else. Situational humor often is of the "You-had-to-be-there" type. It's impossible to recapture everything that happened, and you certainly can't recapture the mood and other intangibles that combined to make the situation really funny. No matter how well you tell the story of what happened, it may just leave people looking at you with a puzzled look, saying "Oh, I see."

Don't be discouraged if this happens to you. Remember that your goal here is not (necessarily) to become skilled at making other people laugh. The goal is to become more adept at observing things that *you* find funny, because this helps sustain your own health, well being, and happiness. It also puts you in a frame of mind that gives you a competitive edge in your work. As you get better at spotting your own humor, you'll also get better at deciding which incidents will and will not be funny to someone else.

A woman explained that she left her parrot in its cage hanging from a nearby tree as she set about mowing the grass in a small cemetery. At a point at which she was some distance from the cage, an elderly woman walked over to one of the recent graves. As she kneeled there, holding flowers and lost in her own grief, she was startled to hear a nearby voice saying, "Helloo-oo." She looked around and found no one, and yet there it was again: "Helloo-ooo." She glanced around again—more frantically this time—and had an uneasy look as she realized she was alone. When she spotted the parrot, she broke out in uncontrollable laughter.[1]

This is a good example of humor that had to be much funnier to both the elderly woman and the grass mower (who eventually came over and heard from the visitor what had just happened). While the story is funny, because we can picture the frightened woman's reaction, it had to be funnier if you were there. It would be difficult to capture in words everything that made her burst out laughing.

Humor Log: Things to Do and Think About

Record your answers to the following in your Humor Log.

On Seeing the Funny Side of Life

1) What does it mean to cultivate a humorous perspective on life?
2) How do humorists view the world? What do they notice that others miss? How do anger, anxiety, or depression make this hard to do?
3) Look around the room and find five things that are blue (square, etc.). These things were in the room all the time, but you never noticed them. How does the same thing occur with humor?
4) Do you agree or disagree with the view that humor is really a form of intellectual play, or play with ideas? Elaborate.
5) Why is it that when you describe to someone else a funny experience you've had, it's generally not as funny to them as it was to you? What does the phrase "you had to be there" mean?
6) The Home Play for the Fifth Habit asks you to record in your Humor Diary the funny things you notice during the next couple of weeks. How will writing them down help develop this habit?

Current Ability to Find Humor in Everyday Life

1) How often do you find tings to laugh at in everyday life (e.g., several times a day, once or twice a day/week/month)?
2) Where are you most likely to notice humor (at work, parties, home, etc.)? Why do you think it happens more there?
3) Who are you most likely to be with when you find things to laugh at? Why does this person help see the funny side of life?
4) What's the funniest thing that has happened to you at work?
5) Think about the day-to-day routines and operations associated with your present job. Find at least two aspects of these routines

which are really pretty absurd or ridiculous, now that you think about it. Also write down why they're absurd.

6) What's the funniest thing that has happened on any prior job?
7) What's the funniest thing that has happened to you in your marriage, or in any other intimate relationship?
8) What funny things have you noticed about the differences in the way men and women react or do things?
9) What impact does your daily mood or stress have on your tendency to notice the funny side of things that happen?
10) What are the conditions under which you are most and least likely to appreciate the humor around you?
11) If you were to pick out one experience in your life which would be a good candidate for *Candid Camera*, what would it be?

Early Development and Influences

1) How good were you at spotting funny incidents during your childhood? Adolescence?
2) What's the funniest thing you can remember happening during your childhood? Adolescence?
3) How good were your mother and father at finding humor in everyday life as you were growing up?
4) Who were the best models you had for learning how to laugh at life (include friends, teachers, and relatives, as well as your parents)? 5) Overall, what has had the greatest impact on your current ability to notice the light side of everyday situations?
6) If you were to give advice to other parents about the value of helping their children learn to find humor in the things that happen in everyday life, what would it be? Why would you give this advice?

GROUP SESSION

Opening Fun Activity

Ask everyone to tell a joke they learned since the last meeting.

Discussion of Home Play for the Fourth Habit

Telling Jokes. What was your experience in starting to tell jokes? How many did you learn? Who did you tell them to? How did they react? How comfortable did you feel doing this? What difficulties did you have, either in remembering or telling the jokes? In what ways are you now better at telling jokes than you were?

Creating Humor. General suggestion: To further develop skills at creating spontaneous verbal humor, look for ambiguous words in your discussion throughout this session. Point them out as they occur. This will help everyone in the group see that the potential for puns and other verbal humor is always present.)

Discuss the following with a partner and then as a group.

1) Bring in examples of word play you noticed in newspapers and on signs, and share them. (Hopefully, they're in your Humor Diary.)
2) How successful were you at noticing ambiguity in conversations?
3) How well did you do at generating puns and other verbal humor?
4) Did you do the exercise in "multiple meanings" every day? Did it help you start thinking in terms of double meanings?
5) Share a couple of daffynitions that you created.
6) Discuss any other aspect of your efforts to improve your verbal sense of humor that you think would be of interest to the group.

Finding Humor in Everyday Life

Draw from any of the issues raised in the above discussion of the Fifth Humor Habit as a starting point for discussion. Each group member should also select one or two suggestions from the Humor Log exercises for detailed discussion within the group.

HOME PLAY

1) Assume that there's a general conspiracy among people to create situations that make you laugh. Go out expecting to find something funny, even in commonplace situations. Ask yourself, "What's funny here?" Or, "What could be funny here?"

2) Keep your little notebook with you at all times. Write funny things down as you see them. Find something to record every day. Look for things at work, at home, in the supermarket, while driving—everywhere you go. Update your Humor Diary daily.

3) Actively remind yourself to maintain a playful frame of mind. This will help you see humor in situations that arise.

4) Continue doing the things you did for the Fourth Habit. This will help set you up to find more unexpected incidents funny.

5) Put up reminders at home, at the office, and in your car to look for humor. Keep a pair of "Groucho glasses" or other props handy as a reminder to be on the lookout for humor.

6) To help sensitize yourself to seeing funny things, change your daily routines. Brush your teeth with the other hand. Put your clothes on in a different order. Wave to people you don't know, etc. Breaking up old behavior patterns helps break up old patterns of thinking, leading you to become more observant of unusual things.

7) Ask friends or colleagues what funny things they have observed, or that have happen to them lately. Specifically ask them about what they find absurd, ridiculous, or bizarre about the policies, rules, and expectations associated with their job, about politics, or any other aspect of life.

8) Make it a point to share the humor you observe with your friends, family, and coworkers.

9) When watching television sit coms, relate funny situations that arise to incidents in your own life. Has anything like this ever happened to you?

10) If you're going through the 7 Humor Habits Program with a group, be prepared to share at the next meeting a funny incident you observed during the week.

11) Remember to stay in touch with your telephone partners.

The Sixth Habit

Take Yourself Lightly
Laugh at Yourself

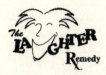

"So many tangles in life are ultimately hopeless that we have no appropriate sword other than laughter. I venture to say that no person is in good health unless he can laugh at himself."

(Gordon W. Allport)

"What is a sense of humor? . . . a residing feeling of one's own absurdity. It is the ability to understand a joke—and that the joke is oneself."

(Clifton Fadiman)

ELEANOR ROOSEVELT ONCE SAID, "**YOU** don't grow up until you have your first good laugh at yourself." The ability to laugh at your own flaws, weaknesses, and blunders has long been recognized as a sign of maturity. And yet it is one of the most difficult aspects of your sense of humor to develop. That is why it is not introduced here until you have progressed in developing other aspects of your sense of humor. You will need the foundation provided by the first five habits if your sense of humor generally disappears when you're the butt of the joke. But you'll be richly rewarded by your efforts in cultivating the Sixth Habit.

We Take Ourselves Too Seriously!

Oscar Wilde offered a keen insight about how to live your life when he said, "Life is too important to be taken seriously." In this paradoxical statement, he did not mean that life doesn't matter. He didn't mean that you shouldn't keep your promises, have integrity, or meet your responsibilities. I believe he meant that if you are serious about everything, the quality of your life suffers.

"What is funny about us is precisely that we take ourselves too seriously." (Reinhold Neibuhr)

Each of us has sensitive areas where it's difficult to lighten up about ourselves. In your case, maybe it's a physical feature. You don't like the fact that you're too skinny, overweight, too tall or short, or that you have a bald spot, dark spots under your eyes, etc. You can joke about most things, but not that! Or maybe you feel clumsy or uneducated, or annoyed by your unassertive style. Perhaps your accent embarrasses you. You will confront these no-laugh zones head-on in working on the Sixth Habit. And you will experience a sense of exhilaration and liberation as you become comfortable with joking about the things that used to simply annoy or embarrass you.

I know a woman who had once been a nun and found any kind of discussion related to sexual issues terribly embarrassing. She helped ease herself out of this by playfully telling her friends, "You know, sex is really a lot like praying . . . Oh God! Oh God!"

As you get better at poking fun at yourself, you will learn to use it to your advantage. President Ronald Reagan's advanced age was a major issue when he ran for reelection. Many felt that he was simply too old for the job. He diffused the issue by poking fun at his age. For example, at one point in the campaign he said, "Well Andrew Jackson left the White House at the age of 75, and he was still quite vigorous. I know, because he told me."

What does it Mean to Take Yourself Lightly?

Have you ever thought about what it means to take yourself lightly? It does not mean:

1) You have a low opinion of yourself.
2) You're putting yourself down.
3) You're incompetent, unprofessional, immature, or irresponsible.
4) You're never serious.

You can take yourself lightly and still hold yourself in high esteem and command respect. In fact, the ability to laugh at yourself generally enhances others' perception of these qualities within you—as long as you don't overdo it! If you direct all your humor at yourself, it will work against you, rather than for you. People will begin to see you as unsure of yourself and as having a poor self-image. And this may lead them to doubt your competence. The key is to show that you are capable of laughing at yourself, not to do it all the time.

You can poke fun at yourself in a way that is either full of fun, acceptance, and positivity, or that's bitter, rejecting, and negative. It's all in the spirit you bring to it. If it comes out of bitterness and self-dislike, you genuinely put yourself down—and lower your self-esteem in the process. In this case, humor makes no positive contribution to your health and well being. But you can also laugh at yourself in a way that is not at all negative—a way that shows that you accept what has happened and are at peace with it.

"There is hope for any man who can look in a mirror and laugh at what he sees." (Anonymous)

In 1988, while running for the presidency, American Vice President George Bush (the first President Bush) was describing his partnership with Ronald Reagan over the preceding eight years. He said, "We've had triumphs. We've made mistakes. We've had sex." The audience exploded with laughter, leaving him no time to correct himself and say "setbacks." Having prepared for just such a moment, however, his comeback was, "I feel like the javelin thrower who won the toss and elected to receive." By poking fun at his embarrassing choice of words, he turned a negative into a positive. If anything, the blunder gained him points in the eyes of the television audience, because it showed he was quick on his feet and could handle people laughing at him.

Taking yourself lightly does mean:

1)   Recognizing that you are not the center of the universe.

In one sense, of course, you are the center of the universe—*your* universe. But in the broader scheme of things, you are a minor figure. Acknowledging this helps many people lighten up about themselves and about minor problems.

When you make a mistake or do something embarrassing, the rest of the world generally doesn't care. So don't brood about it; just accept it for what it is and go on.

2)   Recognizing that your own perspective on things is just one among many that are possible.

This is difficult for many people. You have to "step out of yourself" to really appreciate other perspectives. For example, going to a foreign country helps you see your own country in a new light; you begin to realize that each culture develops its own way of making sense out of the world, and that no single one is more "right" than another.

Do you know why angels can fly?
Because they take themselves so lightly.

In the same fashion, you can broaden your perspective on ways of reacting to life's embarrassing moments, or to some hated personal flaw, by observing how other people adapt to them. Watching other people find a light side of embarrassing moments, or otherwise poke fun at themselves, is very illuminating. It shows you that you don't have to punish yourself for your blunders; you can find a way to laugh at them and move on.

3) Refusing to carry around a sense of heaviness (anger, anxiety, depression, or embarrassment) when you make a mistake or blunder.

My book, *Humor: The Lighter Path to Resilience and Health*, documents how humor and laughter help eliminate these negative emotions in a direct way by providing a cathartic release of pent-up feelings. But learning to take yourself lightly also makes these feelings less likely to occur. It insulates you from them by substituting a positive, upbeat mood that is incompatible with their occurrence. You can't be heavy when you're having a good laugh.

4) Seeing the funny side of your own circumstance or behavior.

When you're good at laughing at yourself, it's just as easy to see the humor of the situation when you commit a blunder as when someone else does. Your ego isn't threatened, so you're free to laugh at the situation itself—even though your own behavior caused the embarrassment. And remember, you're laughing at things you do and that happen to you, not at who you are.

When you can joke about your weaknesses and mistakes, it's a way of admitting that you have them, without letting them hold you down. You develop a kind of upset-free coexistence with them. And once you learn to live with them, you'll find that they simply aren't the problem they used to be.

The serenity prayer of Alcoholics Anonymous says,

"God grant me the serenity to accept the things I cannot change, courage to change the things I can, and wisdom to know the difference."

Alcoholics and drug addicts beginning a 12-Step Recovery Program find very little to laugh at in the early stages of recovery. An early goal of recovery programs is to get the person to simply admit and accept that s/he is an alcoholic or addict. Once this is achieved, it's easier to see humor in some of the crazy things they used to think and do. For example, one recovering alcoholic told me that he never considered it strange to walk across an 8-lane expressway to take a shorter route to get to a liquor store. He now laughs at the crazy things he used to do to get alcohol, or while drunk.

When you laugh at a personal blunder, an oddity of your physical appearance, or a disability you have, you also put those around you at ease. Others initially may feel embarrassed or awkward, but once they see that you can joke about it, they relax. I once knew a man in his 20s who was blind and unmarried. He often wore a T-shirt with the following message on the back: "For a real blind date, call Tom at . . ." and added his phone number. It eliminated the discomfort others often felt around him, got him some laughs—and some dates!

Can You Laugh When You're the Butt of the Joke?

To help assess your own ability to laugh at yourself, think back to situations where you were the butt of the joke. Did you stiffen up, or feel embarrassed or insulted? Sometimes, of course, people disguise real hostility in making you the butt of their jokes. If you feel that's the case, there's no reason to share their laughter. Most of the time, however, it comes out of good-natured fun. And if you can't laugh when others poke fun at you in the spirit of good times, you'll certainly have trouble poking fun at yourself.

> *"If you are willing to make yourself the butt of a joke, you become one of the guys, a human being, and people are more willing to listen to what you have to say."* (Larry Wilde)

The Jewish people have mastered the art of self disparagement. They learned long ago that poking fun at yourself helps you adapt to things that can't really be changed, and invites others to laugh along with you. As you start learning to laugh at yourself, remember that "The not-easily offended shall inherit the mirth."

How to Start Laughing at Yourself

So how do you learn to laugh at yourself, if you've never been good at it? The steps discussed here are presented in an order I've found to be most effective, but if another order works better for you, don't be rigid about sticking to this one. The important thing is to start doing as many of these things as you can. The more you do, the greater and more rapid your progress will be.

Make a List of Things You don't Like about Yourself

Think about the things you don't like about yourself. What are your sensitive zones? Where do your emotional reactions cause you to completely lose your sense of humor? There are two reasons for making this list. First, you need to be specific in targeting aspects of yourself about which you want to lighten up—areas where you're humor impaired. At this point, however, just make the list. Don't try to laugh at yourself yet.

Secondly, for some people, the mere act of creating the list has a surprising effect. A smile creeps onto their face as the list gets longer and longer. By the time they get to the 10th or 15th thing, they see the absurdity of all the things they don't like about themselves.

Divide your list into "heavy" items and more minor ones. Also separating the list into things that can and cannot be changed; this helps you take action when change is possible. It also helps you discover the impact your sense of humor has when you're stuck with an unchangeable situation and have to learn to live with it.

Share One Item on Your List with Someone Every Day, Starting with Minor Items

There is real power in sharing your self-dislikes with others. Some of the barriers to self-acceptance quickly drop just by coming out of the closet of self-dislike and announcing to anyone who'll listen that you're skinny, overweight, a workaholic, and so forth. The mere act of admitting to someone else that you don't like your ears, and that you've always been embarrassed by them (because they stick out), starts breaking down the barriers to acceptance of that part of yourself and to lightening up about them. And you don't even have to joke about them at this point; just express how you feel.

That's why meetings of Alcoholics Anonymous always begin with people saying, "My name is _____, and I'm an alcoholic." They understand the power of publicly admitting something about yourself that's difficult to face up to—and difficult to accept. It helps break down the barriers to overcoming alcoholism.

If you've never experienced what happens when you do this, be sure not to skip this step. You'll see that the more sensitive the area, and the more difficult it is to share, the greater the release you experience from talking about it in public. And the larger the group you share it with, the stronger the effect. But you'll also benefit from sharing it over and over again with one person at a time.

Share Your Blunders and Embarrassing Experiences

Start with past embarrassments. The longer ago they happened, the easier they'll be to discuss. You may even find them funny now. You gradually will get better at discussing these incidents soon after they occur. Start with experiences that are not closely related to your sensitive zones. Then share those that are more difficult to admit.

These incidents often will not be funny to others, because they are "you-had-to-be-there" situations. In some cases, however, they will be funny. One day a nurse walked into a patient's room, and found an older man in the bathroom, bent over the toilet bowl. He had vomited a tremendous amount, and the toilet bowl was looking pretty disgusting. So she flushed it. The man immediately shouted something incomprehensible. By the time he repeated it two or three times, she could finally make it out: "My teeth are in there!" Look for the flushed teeth in your own life, and start telling people about them.

Learn a few Self-Disparaging Jokes

Once you've spent some time with the previous three suggestions, you'll be ready to start poking fun at yourself. An easy way to start is to tell self-disparaging jokes related to whatever you're sensitive about. So be on the lookout for such jokes, and write them down when you hear them. Make it a point to memorize a few. When opportunities arise, tell them to your friends. Any kind of self-put-down joke is a good start, but move quickly to jokes that tap into your own sensitivities. This will help get you used to the feeling of poking fun at yourself and will ease you into coming up with ways of doing so on your own. Be sure to distinguish between doing this in good fun and really putting yourself down.

Try learning a few jokes which put down either your profession or some other group you identify with. If you're a lawyer, for example, you might start with this joke:

> **God and Saint Peter were talking about the problems in heaven. God says, "We're losing money every day. We've got to get things straightened out."**
>
> **Saint Peter asks, "What should we do?"**
>
> **God says, "Get a lawyer to handle it."**
>
> **Saint Peter looks at Him and says, "Now where are we going to find a lawyer up here?"**

If you're constantly embarrassing yourself by forgetting things, practice telling the following joke:

> **A couple who both had recently become concerned about their failing memory were watching TV. A commercial came on and the wife asked her husband if he'd like some ice cream. As she walked out of the room, he said, "Oh, I'd love some. But you'd better write it down, you might forget."**
>
> **"Don't worry," she said, "I can certainly remember that."**

Ten minutes later, she came back with scrambled eggs, and her husband said, "I told you you'd forget the toast!"

Begin Joking about Your Blunders and Things you Don't Like About Yourself

Choose a minor item on your list. Put it on the "front burner" for a day, and look for opportunities to poke fun at it. If this is difficult, start by poking fun at something that doesn't bother you at all (your hair color or lack of hair, your weight, the fact that you wear glasses, etc.). Then proceed to more sensitive areas when it feels right to do so.

"To make mistakes is human; to stumble is commonplace; to be able to laugh at yourself is maturity." (William Arthur Ward)

During the 1992 American presidential race, Ross Perot's ears gave cartoonists a field day. The entire nation roared its approval during one of the presidential debates when Perot spontaneously came up with the line, "I'm all ears." In your case, maybe it's your nose, your double chin, your squeaky laugh, or the way you walk. Be on the lookout for other people's lines that help you poke fun at that part of yourself as you work at coming up with your own.

Recognize that No One is Perfect

An important insight comes when you realize that you're allowed to be imperfect. Every one makes mistakes and has flaws.

A speaker says to his audience, "We've all heard the phrase, 'Nobody's perfect.' If there's anyone here who's perfect, just raise your hand, because I'd really like to meet a perfect person."

No one raises their hand at first. But then he notices a middle-aged man way in the back waving his hand back and forth. "Great!" says the speaker, "We've

finally found a perfect person. Tell me sir, are you really perfect?"

"No, no, no," said the man, "I'm raising my hand for my wife's first husband."

Requiring perfection of yourself on the job, in your relationships, or in developing your sense of humor, sets you up for extra frustration, anger, anxiety, and depression. And that translates into extra stress! You expend incredible energy in connection with your real and imagined weaknesses and blunders. As you carry the tension, anxiety, depression, or anger around, it inevitably starts dragging you down. But as soon as you can say, "Yeah, I blew it!" or "OK, I'm a complete klutz . . . but I'm a lovable Klutz," you feel lighter and act lighter. You come closer to "letting go."

Have a Planned Funny Response for Embarrassing Moments

If you have a funny phrase or action ready for your next embarrassing moment, it will help you react in a lighter manner—even if you don't feel like doing so. You've probably already witnessed some of the standard reactions to embarrassing incidents. They include taking a bow (e.g., after you've dropped your food tray), saying, "For my next trick," or "No applause, please." Or you can be more creative with things like, "And now for something completely different" (from the old Monty Python shows), "You may think that was an accident, but my department is now doing research on reactions to awkward incidents," or "I'm training for the Clumsy Olympics." You're sure to be successful with, "I didn't do it . . . and I'll never do it again."

Maybe you'll feel more comfortable imitating the voice of Elmer Fudd, Donald Duck, Bugs Bunny, Sponge Bob Square Pants, John Wayne, Woody Allen, Presidents George Bush or Barack Obama, or any other famous figure.

A woman who married a man 20 years younger than herself got tired of the same old embarrassing questions

and raised eye brows, so one day she responded with, "Well 20 goes into 40 a lot more than 40 goes into 20."

If the same embarrassing incident occurs often, have a light response ready the next time it occurs. If you're always forgetting things, for example, the next time it happens you might use this line: "My memory is really very good; it's just very short."

Hang around People who are Good at Laughing at Themselves

An excellent way to make progress on the Sixth Habit is to think of the people you know who are good at poking fun at themselves— who don't take themselves seriously all the time. Hang around these people more, and imitate them in any ways that feel comfortable to you. When you see them do something you think would work for you, write it down. Talk to them about how poking fun at themselves makes them feel and why they're good at it, while you aren't.

"If I were given the opportunity to present a gift to the next generation, it would be the ability of each individual to learn to laugh at himself."
(Charles Schulz)

Humor Log: Things to Do and Think About

Remember to record your answers in your Humor Log.

On Laughing at Yourself

1) How would you interpret the phrase, "Life is too important to be taken seriously?"
2) How might taking yourself seriously all the time have a negative effect on your life?

3) What does it mean to "Take yourself lightly, but take your work seriously?"

4) Why is it easier to laugh at embarrassing things that happen to other people than when the same things happen to you?

5) Who among your friends/colleagues is good at laughing at their own flaws or mistakes? Write down a couple of examples you've witnessed that demonstrate this ability.

6) Why do many people experience a sense of liberation and freedom when they first learn to laugh at themselves?

7) How does laughing at yourself produce a feeling of "mastery" or "superiority?"

8) Sometimes laughing at yourself is healthy and adds to self-esteem and your ability to cope. But it also can be unhealthy and reduce your self-esteem and ability to cope. How do these two cases differ?

9) Can being a perfectionist weaken your sense of humor? How?

10) Do you think that men or women are generally better at laughing at themselves? Why do you think this is?

Current Ability to Laugh at Yourself

1) In comparison to other people you know, how good are you at laughing at yourself?

2) Why is this so difficult to do?

3) List in your Humor Log any physical characteristics you have which you don't like, separating them into minor and strong dislikes. 4) List in your Humor Log any behaviors that are typical of you, but that you don't like. Again, distinguish between minor and strong dislikes. Also put a "C" beside those you consider changeable, and a "U" beside those you consider unchangeable.

5) Go back and place a check mark next to the items listed above that you've been able to joke about in the past. As you work on the Sixth Habit, place a check mark next to other items when you manage to poke fun at them.

6) Have any of your sensitive zones had a significant influence on your life over the years? What kind of influence?

7) Is it easier to laugh at your blunders or mistakes when alone or with other people? Why do think that is?

8) List a few embarrassing situations where you have been able to laugh at yourself in public in the past.

9) List a few embarrassing situations where you were unable to laugh at yourself, but wish you could have.

10) In what ways do you feel you have to be perfect? Is it easier or more difficult to poke fun at yourself in these areas?

11) Some people are able to ease into poking fun at themselves by memorizing a few self-putdown jokes. If you were to do this, what kind of joke (in terms of content) would you be looking for (e.g., laughing at one's baldness, eating habits, etc.)?

12) What specific goals would you like to achieve in working on the Sixth Habit?

Early Development and Influences

1) Young children are often very direct and cruel in laughing at others. How good were you at "taking it" when kids laughed at you when you were growing up?

2) What aspects of yourself were you especially sensitive about during your childhood and adolescence? Were you ever able to see humor in connection with these sensitive areas?

3) Has it gotten easier or more difficult to laugh at yourself as you've gotten older? Why do you think that is?

4) Who had the greatest positive and negative influence on your present ability to laugh at yourself?

5) How good were your mother and father at poking fun at themselves?

6) Assume that you would like to help your own children learn the skill of laughing at oneself, so that they'll have access to it as a coping skill when they grow up. What is the most important thing you can do to help them develop this skill?

GROUP SESSION

Opening Fun Activity

Discussion of Home Play for the Fifth Habit

1) How successful were you at noticing funny things this past week?
2) Pair up with a partner and share the funniest incident you've observed since the last meeting.
3) Where did you find the most humor? At home? Work? Elsewhere?
4) What reminders did you use to help remember to look for humor?
5) Did you get better at noticing humor as the week went along?
6) Discuss any difficulties you encountered in sharing a funny event with someone else. Was it as funny to them as it was to you?
7) Take a particular funny incident and describe it to the group—first in a way that captures the essence of what made it funny, then in a way that leaves this out. Discuss these "key" aspects.

Laughing at Yourself

1) Break up into small groups. Describe a situation in your past which was very embarrassing at the moment—and not funny. Discuss how you could have used your sense of humor to lighten up in the situation.
2) Share with a partner a case where you've observed someone really putting themselves down while poking fun at themselves. How might this lower self-esteem and influence others' view of them?
3) Share one of your strongest self-dislikes with a partner. Then discuss how you felt after sharing it.
4) Now imagine that part of yourself in an exaggerated way. Try to make an exaggerated statement about it to your partner. (e.g., "My chin is so pointy, I get stab wounds in my chest if I look at my feet.")

HOME PLAY

Check back with your Humor Log answers in doing this week's Home Play. Do as many of the following as you can (you are not expected to be able to do all of this in a week). This works best if you do items from the top of the list first.

1) Share one item from your "self-dislike" list with someone each day, starting with minor items.
2) Begin sharing blunders, mistakes, and embarrassments.
   a) Keep an eye out for embarrassing situations experienced by others. Think about how you would react if it happened to you.
   b) Ask other people to describe their own funny experiences with personal blunders and embarrassments.
3) Learn a few self-disparaging jokes.
   a) Some of these jokes should have nothing to do with your own sensitive zones. Others should relate directly to your sensitivities. Practice telling them to others.
   b) Seek out comedians who do self-disparaging humor, and spend some time listening to them. Pay attention to your reaction as you listen to or watch self-disparaging humor.
4) Begin joking about your blunders and things you don't like about yourself.
   a) Have a planned funny response for embarrassing moments.
5) Remind yourself that no one is perfect.
   a) Take an area in which you tend to be a perfectionist and find a way to poke fun at it.
6) If you're working on the Sixth Habit with a group, stay in contact with your telephone partners.
7) Record your successes and failures in all of these efforts in your notebook, and then transfer them to your Humor Diary.

The Seventh Habit

Find Humor in the Midst of Stress

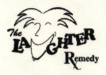

"You cannot prevent the birds of sorrow from flying over your head, but you can prevent them from building nests in your hair."

(Chinese proverb)

"Were it not for my little jokes, I could not bear the burdens of this office."

(Abraham Lincoln)

YOU'VE PROBABLY HEARD THE EXPRESSION, "When life deals you lemons, make lemonade." The term "lemons," in this context, refers to any kind of misfortune. The most important ingredient in making lemonade out of hard times is your sense of humor. Humor can take a sour event in your life and make it sweet(er)—well, at least less sour. By learning to find a light side of any difficult situation, you can transform the hand you've been dealt. So don't let the fact that you're miserable keep you from getting some fun and joy out of life.

My book, *Humor: The Lighter Path to Resilience and Health*, documents the fact that humor has the power to transform a negative mood into a positive one. In the process, it substitutes a frame of mind that is more conducive to finding solutions to the problem of the moment. It also eases your tension and upset and gives you a greater sense of control over your lemons. As you get better at making good lemonade on your worst days, you'll find yourself serving it to others—comfortably and naturally—giving them the same benefits of humor that you enjoy yourself.

"Life is full of misery, loneliness, and unhappiness, and it's all over much too quickly." (Woody Allen)

The French writer and philosopher Voltaire once said, "It is because they can be frivolous at times that the majority of people do not hang themselves." Hopefully, you're not ready to hang yourself because of the stress in your life. But if you're like most people, your stress level has gone up in recent years—especially on your job. The mushrooming growth of the stress management industry provides ample evidence of the increasing stress in our lives. We have seen a proliferation of stress management techniques around the world, including progressive relaxation, deep breathing, meditation, biofeedback, yoga, and more. Amazingly, most of us have completely neglected one of the most effective stress reducers available to us— our sense of humor.

The problem, of course, is that your sense of humor abandons you right when you need it the most. Even if you've consistently done the Home Play for the first six habits, you probably still lose your sense of humor when things start going wrong. The Seventh Habit gives you control over when you use your sense of humor, instead of having it be at the mercy of your mood at the moment. You may even achieve the coolness of the New York hot dog vendor who had a guy aim a gun at him in a robbery attempt. The vender come up with the following line: "Now what do I need a gun for on a job like this? Try selling it to that cop over there." The gunman panicked and ran off—even though there was no cop.

Does Stress Happen to You? Or Do You Create it?

There is a general consensus among psychologists that "you create your own stress." If you've never heard this idea before, it probably makes no sense to you. After all, the victims of the Christmas, 2004 tsunami didn't create the giant wave that took so many lives. The citizens of Haiti did not create the earthquake that devastated their country and their lives in February of 2010. You didn't create the extra work you inherited when your colleague was laid off. You never create the events themselves, but you do determine how stressful they are—depending on how you interpret and react to them.

> *"Perhaps I know why it is man alone who laughs; he alone suffers so deeply that he had to invent laughter."*
> (Friedrich Wilhelm Nietzsche)

If you've ever been in a situation where several people had the same stressors (e.g., cancer, a lost job, or impossible job demands), you've probably noticed that they handle it in very different ways. Some get so angry, anxious, or depressed that their relationships collapse, they lose their effectiveness on the job, and their life falls apart in general. Others have the same initial upset, but quickly accept the reality of the situation and get on to dealing with it.

Bounce-Back-Ability

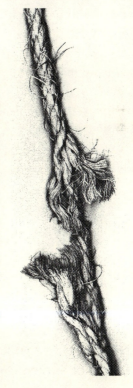

Your sense of humor boosts your resilience by giving you what I call "bounce-back-ability." It helps you bounce back in situations where you feel like you're at the end of your rope—where you'd otherwise succumb. Just as the elasticity of a ball enables it to absorb the energy created by gravity and produce the force necessary to bounce back up against the pull of gravity, your sense of humor gives you the emotional elasticity you need to absorb psychological gravity and bounce back in a more positive direction.

> *"I have seen what a laugh can do. It can transform almost unbearable tears into something bearable, even hopeful."* (Bob Hope)

You will feel the force of psychological gravity pulling you down as you first start trying to use your sense of humor in the midst of stress. It will seem unnatural as you ask yourself, "OK, what's funny about this situation?" Because you know there's absolutely nothing funny about it! But this will pass as you learn to distinguish between the seriousness of the situation and the little things that still could be funny to someone who had the habit of noticing them.

The Importance of Learning to Actively Use Humor

As noted in connection with the First Habit, there are passive and active ways of showing a good sense of humor. You can enjoy humor without ever initiating it yourself. You can laugh at your friends' jokes, listen to TV sit coms, collect *Far Side* or *Dilbert* cartoons, and listen to comedy CDs. These all offer some relief from stress. But you won't always have a friend around when you need a good laugh, and you can't pop a *Saturday Night Live* or *Everybody Loves Raymond* rerun show into your DVD player when things get bad at work. To fully benefit from the stress-reducing power of humor, you need to take control of your opportunities for laughter by coming up with your own humor.

A practical joke was recently played on the leading lady during a live stage performance. A fellow actor had arranged to have the phone unexpectedly ring in the middle of one of her monologues. She picked up the phone, paused a moment, and handed it to her leading man, saying, "It's for you."

How to Practice Finding Humor in the Midst of Stress

This is the most difficult part of your sense of humor to develop. But if you have spent at least a week or two building each of the previous habits, you are now ready to start to lighten up under stress. If you were suffering from Acquired Amusement Deficiency Syndrome (AADS), you've overcome it. You have developed the ability to be more playful and can readily switch back and forth between seriousness and playfulness. You are more sensitized to the funny side of life and have developed the habit of seeking out ambiguities, incongruities, and ironies in your own life. You have even become more expressive of your appreciation of humor; that is, you are laughing more often and more heartily than you did two months ago (although research discussed in Appendix 1 suggests that belly laughter in response to humor is the most difficult habit to change). Your spontaneous verbal wit has improved, and you're better at poking fun at yourself. All of these skills prepare you for what you probably really wanted to do from the beginning—use your sense of humor to cope with stress.

> *"If you don't learn to laugh at trouble, you won't have anything to laugh at when you grow old."* (Ed Howe)

While working on the Seventh Habit, just keep doing what you've been doing. You already have the skills you need to use humor to deal with minor hassles. But those skills probably still don't get you very far under conditions of high stress. The key to success with the Seventh Habit is finding humor in connection with minor hassles and problems first and then moving on to more stressful situations. There are several things you can do to speed up this process.

1) Observe how other people use humor to cope.

Make it a point to watch how others handle stress using humor. If you have friends who are good at this, ask them to share incidents where their sense of humor has helped them cope.

Cancer patients often say that humor and a positive attitude helped get them through their battle with the disease. A cancer patient I know often says, "Anyone who wears hair during the daytime is overdressed." And don't forget about kids. The humorist Erma Bombeck once wrote about a three-year-old cancer patient who had lost her hair, but had a little fuzz reappearing on her head. One day "she observed with curiosity her father's balding head as he bent over to tie his shoe. 'Daddy,' she asked, 'Is your hair coming or going?'"[1]

You can also watch the newspapers for stories about how people use their sense of humor in the midst of stress. For example, after a tornado, a family put up a sign in front of where the house used to be saying, "Gone with the wind." Another tornado victim had his car smashed by a large tree. He put a sign on it saying, "Compact car."

Steve Allen, one of the early *Tonight* Show hosts, was known for his quick wit. In an all-time classic funny TV incident, he described in his book, *How to be Funny*, how he handled an embarrassing situation during his old radio days.

"Jim Moran . . . was on, pushing Persian rugs. He entered, dressed as an Arab, leading an enormous camel. Well, right in the middle of our conversation, the camel began to urinate all over the linoleum floor. Camels have a tremendous capacity to store water, of course, so when they empty their bladders, it takes a while—much longer than for, say, a horse or an elephant.

Anyway, the audience got hysterical. So Jim and I stopped the conversation. The camel went on for about five minutes. The longer he relieved himself, the more the audience laughed. Stagehands came out with buckets and mops to clean up the mess, which was about to spill out into the audience.

After everything was mopped up, the linoleum— originally a dark brown color—was about eight shades lighter, since the waxy buildup, or whatever, had been removed. It had now been reduced to a pale shade of yellow. Suddenly, that transformation struck me funny and I said: 'Say, homemakers, having trouble keeping kitchen floors spotlessly clean?'

The laughter was loud and long."

While you can't expect to match Steve Allen's quick wit at this point, it shows you what's possible, even in the most unpredictable and awkward of situations.

2) Look for a light side of other people's problems (but do not tell them).

It's easier to see a funny side of other people's problems than your own. For example, a woman called a doctor and shrieked that her daughter had swallowed paint thinner. The thought flashed into his mind: "For God's sake, don't let her light a cigarette!" But he kept the idea to himself and simply asked what she had given the child. Humor would never be appropriate in this situation. But the fact that it popped into his mind is a sign of a well-developed sense of humor.

"Everything is funny as long as it happens to someone else."
(Will Rogers)

3) Look for humor in stressful situations in your own past.

Have you ever noticed that things that upset you at the moment often seem funny days or weeks later? The upset disappears with time, allowing your mood to improve to the point where you can see the humor of the situation. Making the effort to see a funny side of past problems will help you find humor in problems as they're occurring.

How many times have you thought, "Some day we'll look back at this and laugh." Why wait? The fact that you say it is a good sign, since it shows that you recognize the potential for humor. But the trick is to learn to laugh at strange, bizarre, incongruous, unexpected, and ironic turns of events as they are happening.

4) Make a list of minor hassles and problems encountered on a typical day. Start looking for humor in these situations.

This may include traffic, annoying colleagues, deadlines, spilling food on yourself, forgetting an appointment, hitting a long check-out line, finding that your child has not done what s/he was supposed to do, etc. To assure success, start off with minor stressors. Be on the lookout for funny things when the next opportunity arises.

Take the initiative in using your joking skills in these situations.

If you find yourself in a hospital for a few days, you might answer a knock at the door by saying, "who's there, friend or enema?" If you're deadly serious about your golf game, and having a bad day, you might lighten things up by saying, "You know, nothing increases my golf score like witnesses."

If you have difficulty doing this, try asking yourself, "What will I find funny about this next month? What's absurd or incongruous here?" Even if you don't find anything funny at the moment, develop the habit of asking the question. Or ask yourself, "What would _____ (name your favorite comedian) find funny about this?"

5) Keep a "lighten-up!" prop handy.

This might be a clown nose, a silly animal nose, a photograph of yourself making a face, your favorite cartoon, etc. (You can use the same props you used for the Second Habit.) You might put up a funny sign in your office. Signs I've seen recently include innocuous ones like "Are we having fun yet?" and "People who think they know everything are particularly annoying to those of use who do." Although crude, my favorite is a bumper sticker which says, "Unless you're a hemorrhoid, get off my ass!" Use these props to help create a mood conducive to finding humor under stress.

> "The one serious conviction that a man should have is that nothing
> is to be taken too seriously." (Samuel Butler)

Keep your props in a place where you know you'll need them (in your pocket, on your desk, in your car, on the refrigerator, etc.). Keeping a cartoon with you at all times works very well for some. It should be a cartoon that brings a grin to your face every time you look at it and symbolizes your commitment to take things a little less seriously. My current favorite cartoon prop shows a woman in a dentist chair, with the usual array of equipment hanging out of her mouth. Her right hand, however, has a firm grip on the male dentist's private parts. The caption reads, "We aren't going to hurt each other, are we doctor?"

Signs Observed on Office Desks

"There will be no crisis next week . . . My schedule is already full."

"Due to current financial constraints, the light at the end of the tunnel will be turned off until further notice."

"You want it by when?" (Shows cartoon figure on floor, laughing.)

---

6) Use funny visual imagery.

Research in the past 20 years has clearly documented the impact of visual imagery on both your mind and body. You can influence your emotional state by conjuring up images associated with a given emotion. Actors do this all the time in order to create a convincing level of communication to the audience.

As you work on the Seventh Habit, practice conjuring up funny visual images as a means of influencing your sour mood. Jot down a few experiences from your past which make you smile every time you think of them. Or create in your own mind a silly or ridiculous image which you will intentionally call forth the next time any regularly-occurring source of stress occurs. This is especially effective when the image involves particular people with whom you often have conflict. The classic approach to this is to imagine the other person in underwear, but use any imagery that works for you. I am especially fond of visualizing people as animals. Each person's body or behavior generally suggests a specific animal to me. The sillier the animal image, the better this works.

7) Practice seeing the glass half-full, instead of half-empty.

This is sure to be a familiar concept to you, but even if you've heard it before, have you ever tried to put it into action? First, decide which kind of person you are. Do you generally see the empty or the full part of the glass? If you focus on the empty part, your first step is to acknowledge your tendency to take positive things for granted, while focusing on the negative. Your task now is to try to adopt an optimistic outlook—and to do so when under stress. Again, begin with minor hassles before trying it with major stressors.

Two older men suffering from the same pancreatic cancer were on the same floor of a hospital and chatted occasionally. One day one of them spotted the other sitting on his bed, head down, looking very depressed. He walked in and asked:

"What's the matter? Why so glum?"

"My doctor just told me that 70% of the people who have what we have don't make it," said the second.

"Oh no, that's not what my doctor said," replied the first. "He said that three out of every 10 survive! And I could be one of those three."

8) Remind yourself that something good often comes out of a bad situation.

I have had many occasions in life where an unwanted outcome turned out to be a blessing in disguise. My entire career in psychology was indirectly due to poor grades in chemistry and calculus during my freshman year of college. At the beginning of my sophomore year, my advisor (a mathematician) saw my grades and asked if I had thought about another major. I had peeked through (but not read) my older brother's psychology text the preceding summer and found it interesting. So I said "psychology," more to avoid the embarrassment of the moment than because of any real interest in pursuing psychology as a major. (If my brother had had an astronomy book, I would have said "astronomy.")

If I had not had such terrible grades my freshman year, I might have continued on to an engineering career—which I would have detested. Had I not failed calculus, I would never have gotten interested in research on humor. I would never have written this book or developed a career as a professional speaker on humor and stress/health. So what seemed like a disaster at the time turned out to have been the best thing that could have happened to me.

When you look back on your own past disappointments and problems, search for unexpected positive outcomes. Then try to do the same thing with problems *as they're happening.* Adopt a wait-and-see attitude when things don't go the way you want them to. Become a "good things" detective, searching for positive outcomes that might occur—while still acknowledging the bad side of the situation.

The following story, often told (in years past) by Dr. Bernie Siegel, illustrates the value of adopting a wait-and-see attitude.

There's a man who has a farm, and his whole livelihood depends on his horse, which plows the fields. One day he's out plowing, and suddenly the horse drops dead. The people of the town say, "Gee, that's tough." And the man says, "We'll see."

A few days later, someone feels sorry for him and gives him a horse. The townspeople say, "What a lucky guy." And the man says, "We'll see." A couple of days later, the horse runs away and everyone says, "You poor guy." And the man says, "We'll see."

A few days later, the horse returns with a second horse, and everyone says, "What a lucky guy!" And the man says, "We'll see." The man had never had two horses before, so he and his son decide to go riding, but the boy falls off his horse and breaks a leg. Everyone says, "Poor kid." And the man says, "We'll see."

The next day, the militia comes into town grabbing young men for the army. But they leave the boy behind, because he has a broken leg. Everyone says, "What a lucky kid!" And the man says, "We'll see."

This story clearly shows that our lives are a constant mix of good and bad things happening. You can get bent out of shape when bad things occur, or wait and see what good will come about as a result of them. You can focus on the negative or anticipate the positive.

Record your answers in your Humor Log.

Humor Log: Things to Do and Think About

On Using Humor to Cope

1) Why is it so hard for most people to keep their sense of humor during stressful times?

2) Describe your own views regarding how humor can help you cope with stress.

3) How do the first six habits help build the foundation for using your sense of humor when under stress?

4) Comment on the idea that situations which are not, in themselves, funny can have a funny side. Describe an example in your own life.

5) People who are regularly exposed to serious injury, death, and dying tend to have a macabre sense of humor, laughing at things that most of us would find horrifying. Why does this occur? What special role does humor serve in these cases?

6) Why does this form of black humor show up in jokes all over the country every time a major disaster occurs?

7) What obstacles to using humor under stress can you expect to encounter if you've never tried this before?

8) Most of us are not very good at solving problems when under stress; we see things more narrowly, and are less creative. How can humor and laughter in the midst of stress lead to more innovative thinking and more effective problem solving?

9) A sense of humor helps you keep everyday hassles and problems in perspective. What does this statement mean?

10) Much of our stress comes from conflicts with other people. With whom do you have the most conflict in your life? How might you use your sense of humor to deal with this conflict?

11) Name two people you know who actively use their sense of humor to cope with stressful events. Describe a specific case where you've seen them initiate humor in a difficult situation.

12) Considering the different skills you've developed while working

on the first six habits, which ones do you expect to be especially helpful to you in dealing with stress?

13) Describe two conflicts which often come up at work or at home. How might you use humor to help diffuse the conflict in the future?
14) Why should an active use of humor be more effective than a passive enjoyment of humor in helping you cope with stress?
15) Can you think of any reasons why parents might hesitate to use a joking remark in front of their children in the midst of a family conflict? How could these reasons be satisfactorily overcome?

Current Ability to Find Humor in the Midst of Stress

1) Disregarding your use of humor, how well do you generally cope with stressful events in your life?
2) How would you describe your present skills at finding a light side of a) mildly and b) highly stressful situations?
3) Describe a recent stressful event which best demonstrates your present use (or lack of use) of humor to cope.
4) Has your ability to use humor to cope already improved as a result of your efforts at the Home Play for the first six humor habits? If so, how?
5) Have you ever used humor in difficult situations to hide from the problem, or deny it? If so, what needs to be changed in order to use humor in a positive, constructive manner?
6) What are your goals in working on the Seventh Habit?

Early Development and Influences

1) How much stress was there in your family as you were growing up (both during childhood and adolescence)?
    a) What was the most common source of stress during each period?
2) What was the most difficult thing to adjust to in connection with a) parents, b) brothers/sisters, c) friends, d) school and e) dating?

3) Can use remember ever using humor to cope while growing up? If so, how?

4) Think of an example from both your childhood and adolescent years of a stressful situation in which you would like to have come up with a humorous remark to handle a problem, but were unable to do so. How might you have used your sense of humor to deal with this?

5) Did your parents ever react negatively to some effort at humor on your part in the midst of a family conflict? Positively? Describe the situation and their reaction.

6) How good were your parents at using humor in the midst of family conflicts? Give an example which demonstrates both your mother's and father's use (or lack of) use of humor.

7) List any other significant adults during your childhood who showed a good sense of humor in the midst of stress.

GROUP SESSION

Opening Fun Activity

Discussion of Home Play for the Sixth Habit

1) Share with a partner your efforts in learning to laugh at yourself. Describe specific cases where you were and were not successful.
2) If time permits, also share with a partner
   a) Your list of things you don't like about yourself.
   b) Whether you shared items from this list with others during the week and whether you were able to poke fun at any of them.
   c) Your success at finding humor in a blunder or embarrassing event.
   d) Obstacles you encountered in trying to poke fun at yourself.
   e) A self-disparaging joke that you learned.
3) Discuss with a partner the idea that you can take yourself lightly, while taking your work and responsibilities seriously.

Finding Humor in the Midst of Stress

1) Discuss any of the issues raised in the Humor Log exercises for the Seventh Habit.
2) Why is it so much easier to find a light side of things in the midst of someone else's stress?
3) Discuss which of the habits each group member thinks will be most useful in using humor to cope.
4) Share (if possible) an occasion where you were successful in using humor to cope with a difficult moment.
5) Describe a specific stressful situation from your own experience, preferably one that occurs often now. The group should discuss ways in which you could use humor to lighten up in that situation.
6) Discuss why it is so difficult to keep your sense of humor when you're having a bad day.
7) If you're going through the Program with co-workers, break up into small groups and try to come up with a lighter way to respond to a stressful situation facing most employees present.

HOME PLAY

In general, just keep doing what you've been doing in connection with each of the first six habits. Remember, you are not expected to do all of the suggestions included below. Find the ones that work best for you. Record your ideas and observations in your Humor Diary.

1) Make a list of commonly occurring hassles and problems. Be determined to find a way to maintain a lighter attitude when these come up, while remaining committed to handling the problem. Give special attention to sources of stress at home and at work.

2) Think about what it means in these particular situations to see the glass "half full" instead of "half empty."

3) Ask friends to help you find a light side of difficult situations.

4) Practice finding humor in connection with other people's problems (but keep it to yourself).

5) Look for humor in past stressful situations of your own.

6) Develop the habit of asking, "What will I find funny about this next week?"

7) Keep a prop handy which reminds you to "Lighten Up!"

8) When your stress centers around your boss, or some other person to whom you may not feel free to fully express yourself, visualize him/her in some ridiculous way (e.g., as a pig oinking, a sheep bleating, in underwear, etc.) the next time a conflict comes up.

9) Think of a silly behavior or statement you can use to help maintain a playful outlook the next time a common problem arises.

10) Ask yourself, "How would Charlie Chaplin (or your favorite comedian) react in this situation?" Imagine you're that person.

11) Keep track of incidents where you are able to be more playful or find a light side of a difficult situation. Don't worry about how funny it is. Note even minor examples.

12) Follow as many suggestions as you can in the section on "How to practice finding humor in the midst of stress."

13) Remember to contact your phone partners this week. Be sure to support each other's efforts at using humor to cope.

INTEGRATE THE HABITS INTO EVERYDAY LIFE

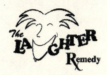

"If you want to rule the world, you must keep it amused."
(Ralph Waldo Emerson)

"I try to think of humor as one of our greatest . . . national resources that must be preserved at all costs."

(James Thurber)

IF YOU'VE SPENT A WEEK or two building up each of the 7 Humor Habits discussed in this book, you've made a tremendous amount of progress, and you're now ready to put all the habits together and actively use humor to cope. You should be aware, however, that as you've put different aspects of your sense of humor on the "front burner" from one week to the next, you may have lost some of the gains made on earlier steps. You now know that it takes more than a week or two to make the skills associated with each habit a permanent part of your personality—your habitual approach to relating to people and living life generally. By taking a little time now to reexamine where you stand with each habit, you'll see which areas of your sense of humor still need more work and can give them special attention.

During this follow-up period, you're asked to consciously work on all of the steps at the same time. This will further strengthen each of the skills and habits you've been developing, helping to put them on "automatic pilot." That is, it will make them available when you need them, with no real effort on your part.

Assessment of Your Progress

You will find below a series of questions related to each of the habits in this Humor Habits Program. You will be asked to think about the progress you've made on each of the habits and how these skills or habits have influenced other aspects of your life. Answer these questions, and use the information gained to decide for yourself where the strong and weak parts of your sense of humor now lie. Do that now, before moving on to the next section below. Write your answers in your Humor Log. Writing these down (instead of just thinking about them) gives you a sharper and more detailed sense of just how much progress you've made.

The First Habit

1) Compare the extent to which you now build outside sources of humor into your life to your pattern before starting this program. How much more daily exposure to humor do you now have?
2) Answer the same question specifically with respect to television, movies, print cartoons, stand-up comedy, and funny friends.
3) How has immersing yourself in humor for the past few months influenced your sense of humor?
4) What insights about the nature of your sense of humor have you had as a result of this immersion in humor?

The Second Habit

1) What progress have you made in overcoming Terminal Seriousness?
2) In what situations do you still find it difficult to adopt a lighter, more playful attitude?
3) Given your experience with this Program, how important do you now think playfulness is for developing your sense of humor?

4) If you've made the effort to adopt a more playful style at work, how successful has this been? How is it now being received?

5) If you've made the effort to be more playful in your personal relationships, how would you describe its effect?

The Third Habit

1) Describe how your laughter has changed as you've gone through this program—both in terms of how often and how heartily you laugh. Research has shown this habit to be the most resistant to change. Was this the case for you?

2) How important a role does an occasional belly laugh play in managing your mood and helping you cope with stress?

The Fourth Habit

1) Compared to before you started the 7 Humor Habits Program, how often do you now tell jokes or funny stories?

2) In what ways are you now a better joke teller than you used to be?

3) To what extent has joke telling helped you deal with stress?

4) How have your skills at creating your own verbal humor improved?

5) At present, what is your most common way of playing with language (e.g., puns, exaggeration, nonsense, etc.)?

6) To what extent does coming up with your own spontaneous puns or other verbal humor now help you cope with stress?

The Fifth Habit

1) Describe your progress in finding humor in everyday life situations at work, at home and elsewhere.

2) Where have you been most and least successful at finding a funny side of things?

3) To what extent has your ability to find humor in everyday life circumstances helped you cope with stress?

The Sixth Habit

1) How much improvement have you shown in your ability to laugh at yourself as a result of this program?
2) List the areas where you've been most and least successful in learning to poke fun at yourself.
3) To what extent has being able to laugh at yourself helped you cope with stress?

The Seventh Habit

1) How much progress have you made in using your sense of humor to cope with stress as a result of this Humor Habits Training Program?
2) Which of the habits has been most useful in helping you cope?
3) Which habit would you like to continue working on to get even better at using humor to cope?
4) In what areas of your life have you been most/least successful in using your sense of humor to cope?

Putting it All Together

If you've done the Home Play for each of the 7 Humor Habits during the past two to four months, you've strengthened the weaker areas of your sense of humor and are now ready to put it all together and develop a well-balanced and mature sense of humor. You're ready to actively use your sense of humor to cope. Use the next week or two to practice some of the skills associated with each habit every day. You'll soon be able to forget about having to actively look for opportunities to use the various habits. They'll just occur to you automatically. This is the point at which you know that your sense of humor will always be there to help you cope. It will serve you as a life preserver when you're drowning emotionally. If at all possible, *spend two weeks on this final part of the Program*. This will help assure that you internalize all the gains you've made.

In addition to helping you cope, humor and laughter will now also help prevent stress from occurring. So you can *start thinking of your sense of humor as a stress deodorant*! If you're lucky, one application in the morning will get you through the day. Chances are, however, that with your life, you'll need repeated applications all day long. You now have the skills to make this happen.

Use your Humor Diary to keep a daily record of the number of times you use skills associated with each habit each day (as discussed below). Be sure to do this. It will help assure that you do the final Home Play, and will show you which set of humor skills and habits you seem to be most comfortable with. It will also reveal which humor habits you draw on when you're under stress.

Take the Sense of Humor Post-Test

After finishing this week or two of putting it all together, take the post-test (identical to the pre-test) provided in Appendix 3. If you have been completing the 7 Humor Habits Program with a group, and the group is having eight meetings, complete the post-test prior to the 8th meeting so that you can discuss it in the group. Do not consult your answers on the pre-test until after you've completed the post-test. Then compare your pre- and post-test scores. Describe in your Humor Log any insights you gain about your progress after comparing these scores. Pay attention to specific items on the humor test, in addition to the total scores. If you've been going through the 7HH Program alone, make it a point to discuss these differences with some of your friends or co-workers.

Group Session

Opening Fun Activity

Discussion of Home Play for Step 7

1) Share a successful and unsuccessful attempt at lightening up in the midst of stress.
2) Humor can be thought of as an attitude, a way of looking at things which keeps you from being overwhelmed by the stressful event. Discuss this idea in light of specific stressors you've encountered.
3) Describe to the group a specific stressful situation that has come up since the last session. Give the group the task of deciding how you could have used humor in this situation, or reacted in a lighter and more effective way.
4) How successful were you at seeing the glass "half full," instead of "half empty?"
5) How successful were you at finding a funny side of other people's problems? Did this help you lighten up when you had a problem?
6) What props or cartoons did you use to help you maintain a lighter attitude in difficult situations?
7) Was it easier to use humor to deal with stress at home or at work?
8) Which steps of this Program were most useful in helping you cope with stress? Which humor skills did you use most often?
9) All things considered, how has this Program influenced the general level of stress in your life?

Progress in Improving your Sense of Humor

1) Share your feelings about how you've benefitted from this Program.
2) In what areas have you made the most/least progress in improving your sense of humor?
3) If you've already completed the post-test, share the results with a partner. Discuss difference from your pre-test for each habit, and communicate any insights you gained from the post-test.

HOME PLAY

This final *two-week period* allows you to consolidate the gains you've made and make them an integral part of yourself. Practice all of the habits you've worked on. Give special attention to the areas you consider your weak points. Refer back to the Home Play related to those areas to which you want to give extra attention.

Use the daily log on the next page (or do the same thing in the personal Humor Log you've been using) for a two-week period to record the number of times you use any of the skills associated with Habits 2-6. *Indicate in the parentheses provided how many of those efforts at humor helped you cope with a difficult or stressful situation.* For example, if you initiated some form of verbal humor five times on a given day, and it really helped you cope in two situations, you would fill in the blank as follows: 5 (2) . Do this every evening before going to bed. Recording these will clarify to you which parts of your sense of humor are serving you best as a coping tool.

Once you've completed this two-week log of your daily use of different humor skills, spend some time analyzing the patterns that emerge. If this two-week period is typical of your everyday life, you now have a basis for stating which parts of your sense of humor are more and less well developed. You can also see what does and does not work for you in terms of the components of your sense of humor that help you cope with life stress.

> **There's this guy who's a big shot in guns. And yet he gets fired several times a day. He works for the circus, getting shot out of a cannon. Finally, he decides he's had it, and he quits. His boss says to him sadly, "I hate to see you go. We'll never find another guy of your caliber."**

Don't worry about the fact that some humor habits showed up frequently, while others didn't show up much at all. Even though you've now spent a lot of time and energy working on all of these basic humor skills, it's important to remember that we all have our own natural comfort levels with certain kinds or styles of humor,

Frequency of Use of Humor Habits/Skills

Week 1

	Habit 2	Habit 3	Habit 4	Habit 5	Habit 6
Mon.	_____	_____	_____	_____	_____
Tues.	_____	_____	_____	_____	_____
Wed.	_____	_____	_____	_____	_____
Thurs.	_____	_____	_____	_____	_____
Fri.	_____	_____	_____	_____	_____
Sat.	_____	_____	_____	_____	_____
Sun.	_____	_____	_____	_____	_____

Week 2

	Habit 2	Habit 3	Habit 4	Habit 5	Habit 6
Mon.	_____	_____	_____	_____	_____
Tues.	_____	_____	_____	_____	_____
Wed.	_____	_____	_____	_____	_____
Thurs.	_____	_____	_____	_____	_____
Fri.	_____	_____	_____	_____	_____
Sat.	_____	_____	_____	_____	_____
Sun.	_____	_____	_____	_____	_____

while we feel less comfortable or natural with others. You've made the effort to strengthen all the skills, but certain habits are now really ingrained into you, while others still require conscious effort.

You may have discovered your own natural sense of humor. Don't worry about the fact that your daily use of different kinds of humor is not balanced. The important thing is that you find at least one set of humor skills and habits that get fully internalized into your daily style of interaction. This one set of humor habits (two or more is icing on the cake) will probably turn out to be the one that really helps you cope with life's daily burdens. You can consider the 7 Humor Habits Program a resounding success if you have wound up with one or two sets of humor skills that are finely honed and serve you well in the midst of stress.

HOME PLAY FOR THE MONTHS AHEAD

You can now see that it takes time and effort to change your old habits relating to humor and laughter. You've made progress, but you'd probably like to make more. One way to do so is to let this book sit for a few months—or as long as a year—and then start back at the beginning, repeating at least some of the Home Play for each of the humor habits. You'll find that the habits will become more firmly entrenched into your personality the second time around.

Another way to continue benefiting from the Program is to simply extend this two week period of "putting it all together" into the months and years ahead. Make it a point periodically to think about whether you're being as playful as you want to be, making enough effort to play with language and laugh at yourself; and be sure to actively look for humor—especially on your bad days.

Like any set of skills, if you don't use them, they atrophy. So you'll need to make a commitment to continue building humor into your life, both by creating it yourself and looking for it in everyday life. To help sustain the development of your sense of humor, create a Mirth Aide Kit, using the props, CDs, cartoons, and anything else you've collected that helps you laugh when you're having a bad day. Keep a separate kit at home and at work.

Consider putting this book aside for a year and going through the Program again. If possible, do it with a partner. And remember to make it fun, not work.

In the months ahead, use your sense of humor to provide a daily emotional cleansing. You cleanse your body every day by washing it, and you nourish it by eating. You keep it in good condition to perform physical tasks by exercising it. You nourish your mind by reading, listening to the news, and talking to people. But what daily activities do you engage in to cleanse and nourish your emotions? Establishing loving relationships with others is crucial, but you also need a regular means of letting go of the negative emotions that accumulate on high stress days. Humor and laughter help you manage your daily mood, as well as the mood of other important people in your life.

Humor helps you take control of your emotional state, even if you're powerless to control the situation itself. In taking control of your frame of mind, you are better able to take the necessary steps to manage the problems that cause you daily stress. Your sense of humor provides an emotional release that is just as cleansing as the soap on your body. It is nourishment for your soul. And when you experience this cleansing yourself, you'll inevitably pass it on to others. So do what you can to put more MIRTH ON EARTH.

It's All in Your Hands

An old tale describes a man who for many years was known across the land for his great wisdom. He would go from town to town and give people advice about their love life, their job, raising a family—about any problem at all. He's a sage, and he's loved in every town he goes to—except one. There are two men in this town who are jealous of all the attention and respect he gets. So they try to make him look bad, even though they, themselves, could never achieve his level of wisdom.

The wise man is coming to their town the next day. And one of the men comes to the other and says, "You know, I've finally figured out a way to make him look bad." And his friend says, "Well, what are we going to do this time?" The first says, "Well, I'm going to be the first one in line tomorrow. And I'm going to say, 'Wise man, many of us in this town think you've lost your wisdom. In fact, we think you're getting senile. To prove your wisdom once and for all, just answer the following question.'"

So his friend says, "Well, what's the question?" "Well, I'm going to have a little butterfly in my hands, and I'm going to ask him whether the butterfly is alive or dead. If he says it's dead, I'll just open up my hands, and it'll fly away. But if he says it's alive, I'll just gently crush my hands together, and everybody will see a dead

125

butterfly." His friend gets really excited and says, "So no matter what he says, he's going to be wrong."

Well, they couldn't wait until the next day's confrontation. Everything goes according to plan, and they are the first ones in line. There are several hundred people there, and when the wise man shows up, the second man causes a big ruckus to get everyone to gather around. The first man says, "Wise man, many of us in this town think you've lost your wisdom. In fact, we think you're getting senile. To prove your wisdom once and for all, just answer the following question." And he put his hands up and said, "Is the butterfly in my hands alive or dead?"

The wise man doesn't even hesitate. He looks him in the eye and says, "The answer to that question is very simple. It's all in your hands . . . It's your choice."

Think of the butterfly as your sense of humor. You know from your own experience that your sense of humor is easily crushed by the stress from your job, relationships, the current economic crisis, health problems, the constant threat of terrorism—by all the areas in your life where things can go wrong. But if you nurture it and use the 7 Humor Habits Program to build it up, it can also help you fly. It can carry you to heights that make it easier to cope with anything life throws your way. It can provide you with joy and a love of life even in the midst of hard times. It can give you a sense of control over your daily mood and leave you in a frame of mind that is better equipped to handle problems effectively. It can help you cope!

This book and its companion, *Humor: The Lighter Path to Resilience and Health,* provide you with all the incentive you should need to make the effort to improve your sense of humor. Whether or not you allow this playful butterfly to die or develop and thrive is all in your hands . . . It's your choice.

Appendix 1

Research Documenting the Effectiveness of the 7 Humor Habits Program

Summary for the General Reader
The Program Works!

Several studies have shown that this Humor Habits/Skills Training Program does work. *People who spend eight weeks doing the Home Play do improve their sense of humor and do improve their ability to use humor to cope with stress.* All of the studies completed used (at least part of) the SHS scale included in Appendix 3, and consistent boosts in this measure of sense of humor have been demonstrated for individuals ranging in age from late teens (college students) to senior citizens (with an average age of 82). So, it's never too late for *you* to improve your sense of humor.

These studies have also shown that completing the *7 Humor Habits Program reduces stress and negative mood* (including depression) and *increases one's daily positive mood* (including cheerfulness and a general playful attitude; remember that a playful attitude is the basic foundation for your sense of humor). The Program has also been shown 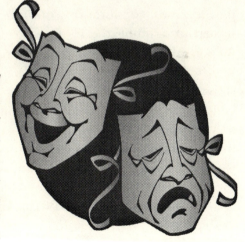 to *increase optimism, a perceived sense of control over one's internal states and degree of satisfaction with one's life.* All of these additional benefits of the Program clearly go a long way toward boosting one's emotional resilience in facing the mounting challenges we face in a stressed-out world.

Detailed Discussion

Studies of the impact of the 7 Humor Habits Program have used a broad range of types of participating subjects and widely varying assessment measures. Most studies have used individuals meeting in weekly group sessions, although this is not essential for the success of the Program. All studies have used one or more parts of the Sense of Humor Scale (SHS) presented in this book, along with other measures. Most of these additional measures were standard measures of stress and positive or negative emotion, but other measures were also used, reflecting the particular concerns of the researchers doing the study.

The exact procedures used in these studies also differed, although all followed the general guidelines of the Humor Log exercises and Home Play suggestions provided in this book. It should be remembered that the 7HH Program was designed with this flexibility in mind. Most people find that the Humor Log and Home Play exercises presented here are excessive. This was done purposefully so that people can pick and choose those activities and exercise that they feel most comfortable with. The key is to be doing something related to building the habits each week. As long as the activity supports the development of a given habit, it does not matter exactly which activity is engaged in. Of course, the greater the number of activities done, the greater the progress to be expected. (It should be noted that—to my knowledge—none of these studies attempted to assess the extent to which participating subjects actually engaged in the exercises and activities proposed to them. So it is impossible to determine the impact of amount of effort exerted in developing the habits on the results discussed here.)

All of these studies tested what was previously referred to as the 8-Step Humor Skills Training Program. The name of the program has been changed to the 7 Humor Habits Training Program, but the actual program tested in those studies is the same as the program presented here. The word "skill" has simply been changed to "habit."

The first study used senior citizens (mean age = 82 years) living in a retirement community in the USA (New Jersey).[1] One group spent 8 weeks going through the Program, and actively worked on improving humor skills using portions of the Home Play provided for each step. In addition to discussing Home Play from the previous week, these sessions included games, joke/story telling and a lot of laughter. The other group spent the entire (one-hour) meeting time watching comedy videos for the same 8-week period (passive exposure to humor). The specific videos watched were selected by participating subjects. The passive group sessions also included games and friendly banter.

While the two groups showed similar coping abilities at the beginning of the study, the active humor training group scored significantly higher than the passive humor group on the "humor under stress" subscale of the Sense of Humor Scale or SHS (the scale that accompanied the Training Program—also presented in this book) and two additional measures of coping with stress in general (without consideration of humor). These included the Pain and Distress Scale (PADS) and a single item self-report question, "In general, I am able to cope well with daily stresses." (The other parts of the SHS were not administered.) Since the average of subjects participating in this study was 82, this finding suggests that you're never too old to improve your sense of humor and use it to cope with life stress.

In an Austrian study, a group of adults completed the Program with weekly meetings and completion of Home Play by the experimental group.[2] There was also a one-month follow-up in this study. Three additional groups were included. The first group completed the Humor Training in the usual fashion. A second received only a theoretical discussion of the training during weekly meetings, but did not actually practice the humor habits. A third discussed socially relevant topics at the meetings (but not humor), and a fourth just completed the various measures on the same timetable as the other groups. The training yielded a significant increase in all six subscales of the SHS, along with an increase in both playfulness and positive mood (McGhee's scales). These increases were still present a month after completion of the Program. The training also produced a significant increase in a separate Coping Humor Scale[3] and decreases in both the seriousness and bad mood scales of the State Trait Cheerfulness Inventory.

Amazingly, the group that just got together weekly and discussed humor every week also improved their scores on both the SHS and the Coping Humor Scale. Their playfulness and positive mood also increased. So even though they were not specifically trained in building humor skills, their sense of humor improved. The reason for this improvement may lie in the lesson learned in the Swiss study (discussed next). The researchers in that study learned that subjects who were just meeting regularly to watch funny videos and talk about humor actually met among themselves to talk about humor and what they were doing in the study. Since they were clearly putting humor "on the front burner" during the study, they may well have been practicing some of the humor habits on their own without being asked to do so. It should be noted, though, that the gains within this group that presumably merely discussed humor at the weekly meetings were not as great as the gains for the group actively working on building stronger humor habits.

A Swiss study tested the Program using four non-student adult groups (mean age = 47 years).[4] Three different experimental groups met every two weeks for two-hour sessions. The fourth group was a control group which only met three times to take the same tests the experimental groups took. Of the experimental groups, one completed Home Play activities and exercises for each habit between the eight sessions. A second group participated in the same kind of discussions within session meetings, but was not asked to do any Home Play activities. Thus, the second group received similar training within meetings, and presumably only differed in the extent to which they practiced the humor skills associated with each step between bi-weekly meetings. A third group received passive exposure to humor during the eight meetings, but had no form of humor training.

Both of the humor training groups showed a significant increase in scores on McGhee's Sense of Humor Scale from the pre- to post-test, as well as on a measure of trait cheerfulness. These changes were sustained at a two-month follow-up test. It is worth noting that the same sustained improvement in SHS scores occurred for the two humor training groups when peers rated subjects' sense of humor using the SHS. Surprisingly, the passive humor group showed an improvement in SHS scores comparable to that shown by the two training groups. The researchers learned after the completion of the study, however, that this group had gotten together on their own several times between sessions to discuss humor. This suggests that even the regular passive exposure to humor as part of a study may have been enough to stimulate subjects' interest in taking a more active effort to improve their sense of humor.

The humor training sessions boosted the level of positive mood and playfulness within each of the eight sessions. This is to be expected, given the fun focus of the sessions. There was no change, however, in positive mood and playfulness between the pre- and post-test. Finally, each of the humor training groups (and only these two groups) showed a significant increase in a measure of life satisfaction as a result of the training.

The most thorough test of the 7 Humor Habits Training Program to this point was completed using an Australian sample of adults (mean age = 37 years)[5]. All subjects completed a series of tests two weeks prior to the beginning of the study, at the end of eight weekly sessions, and three months after the final session. The experimental group received weekly one-hour skill training sessions (incorporating Home Play for each habit) for eight weeks, while a "social group" met for the same eight weeks for tea and "humorous banter," but no humor training of any kind. A third non-treatment control group met three times for the sole purpose of taking the full set of measures.

Significant changes in scores on the measures listed in the table on the next page were obtained between pre-test and post-test, and were sustained or continued to increase/decrease at the three-month follow-up (no significant change was found for either control group in any of these, unless otherwise specified).

This study, then makes a convincing case for the effectiveness of the 7 Humor Habits Training Program in boosting specific (self-rated) humor skills—including a significant improvement in the ability to use humor to cope with stress—and a more positive humor style (affiliative and self-enhancing humor). In the process, it strengthened a more playful, positive and optimistic mood, while reducing depression, stress and negative affect in general. It also boosted a perceived sense of self-efficacy and a perceived sense of control over one's internal states. This latter finding is especially important in connection with research on emotional intelligence, which suggests that the ability to effectively manage one's emotions is a central component of emotional intelligence.

It is also noteworthy that the Humor Training Program had no impact on the Laughing at Oneself subscale of the SHS or the Self-Defeating Humor Style[6]. This supports the notion that learning to poke fun at yourself may be the most difficult humor skill to acquire.

Upon completion of all the tests at the three-month follow-up, subjects were asked to complete an evaluation form regarding the program as a whole. Ninety percent of the Training Group indicated that they did feel more able to deal with stressful events in the three months following the completion of the program (10% were unsure). Also, and most importantly, 95% of them said that they *had* used the humor skills learned in the sessions during those three months.

Two researchers have tested the effectiveness of the 7HH Program with college students. In one study, students from two different German universities completed both the SHS pre- and post-tests via e-mail.12 They were also sent via e-mail selected Humor Log exercises and Home Play activities that they were asked to complete. Once the study started, they were sent two e-mails per week, and the 7HH Program was completed in four weeks, instead of eight. While all subjects were reported to show increased SHS scores as a result of the Program, no statistical analyses were completed of the results, so it is difficult to assess the actual impact of this training program. Increased playfulness and positive attitudes were also noted as a result of the Program, but—again—no data analyses were reported.

One faculty member at an American university (discussed below) has included asking students to go through then 7HH Program in the normal fashion as part of the requirements of a college course

Findings from the Australian Test of the 7 Humor Habits Program

Increased

Humor under stress – SHS subscale
Coping Humor Scale – See reference 3
Verbal humor – SHS
Finding humor in everyday life – SHS
Enjoyment of humor – SHS
(No analyses were run on total SHS scores.)
Affiliative humor – See reference 6
Self-enhancing humor – See reference 6
Playful attitude – McGhee's scale
Positive mood – McGhee's scale
Positive affect – Positive & Negative Affect Scale[7]
Perceived self-efficacy – Generalized Self-Efficacy Scale[8]
Perceived control of internal states – PCOISS[9]
Optimism

Decreased

Stress – Perceived Stress Scale[10]
Stress – Depression Anxiety Stress Scale[11]
Depression – See reference 11
Negative affect – See reference 7

No Significant Change

Laughter – SHS
Laughing at yourself – SHS
Self-defeating humor – See reference 6
Use of aggressive humor – See reference 6
Anxiety – See reference 11

on humor and therapy. He has reported that even completion of a very limited number of Humor Log exercises and Home Play activities while devoting one week to each habit in the context of a college course was sufficient to produce significant improvement in each of the seven habits except for amount of laughter.13 A significant improvement was also shown in cultivating a playful attitude, maintaining a more positive mood.

Reduced Clinical Depression, Anxiety and Stress

While the 7 Humor Habits Training Program was not designed as a clinical tool, it is worth noting that a consistent finding across numerous humor studies (these are reviewed in my book, Humor: The Lighter Path to Resilience and Health) is that exposure to humor is an effective means of elevating one's emotional state or mood. We are more likely to find or initiate humor ourselves when already in a positive mood, but outside sources of humor can also pull us into a more upbeat, positive and optimistic mood.

The ultimate test of humor's power in this respect would be with individuals diagnosed with clinical depression. Clinically depressed people have a chronic inability to experience pleasure, joy and aliveness; they have a very negative, pessimistic view of their future. Since humor and laughter have been shown to stimulate known pleasure centers in the brain and trigger the experience of joy, humor may well be able to support the ability to pull oneself out of severe depression. Numerous studies of humor have documented the power of humor to reduce or help manage depression.14 So training effective humor skills in depressed individuals should be an effective means of helping them manage their depression.

Three studies have demonstrated that the completion of the 7HH Program does reduce clinical depression. For example, at the time of the pre-test (three weeks prior to the first humor training session) in the Australian study, 38% of the subjects in the experimental group met the criteria for clinical stress and depression (using the Depression, Anxiety and Stress Scale); 24% met it for clinical anxiety. By the post-test this percentage had dropped to 9.5%, 9.5% and 0% for depression, stress and anxiety, respectively. At the three-month follow-up, the percentage was 4.8%, 0% and 0% respectively.6 This suggests that this skill development program may be worthy of investigation as a clinical tool.

Two such studies have been completed in Germany. One was specifically designed to determine whether a humor training program could boost the effectiveness of a standard program for the treatment of depression. A small group (11) of clinically depressed patients were guided through an abbreviated (four week) version of the 7HH Program, while still receiving the standard treatment for depression.15 This standard treatment included a combination of depression-related drugs and consultation with a therapist.

There were two meetings per week, with each meeting devoted to one of the humor habits. While this shortened version of the program did significantly boost these patients' appreciation/enjoyment of cartoon humor (in comparison to a similar patient group who received no humor training), it did not add to the effectiveness of the regular treatment program. Nor did it produce an increase in scores on the SHS (actually, there was an increase, but not a significant one). Since every other assessment of the 7HH Program has demonstrated improvement in this measure of sense of humor, it seems likely that four weeks is simply not enough time for the Program to have a meaningful impact on sense of humor—especially among severely depressed individuals. This is not enough time to actually build the humor skills composing the Program as regular habits—as an integrated part of their personality and approach to dealing with everyday life.

Finally, another German study also examined the ability of the 7HH Program to boost depressed patients' humor abilities.16 The goal of this study was to see if boosting humor skills could help elevate patients' mood and enable them to use humor to cope. It was viewed by the researchers as a pilot or exploratory study, since only eight subjects were used. They did find, however, that completion of the program in the usual eight-week time frame produced a significant improvement in cheerfulness and decreased seriousness. Mood also showed a significant improvement within most of the weekly sessions.

The Program also produced a significant increase in extent of agreement with these questionnaire items:

"Humor helps me cope with difficulties."

"Humor is helpful in my particular situation."

Consistent with this, the Program yielded a marginally significant increase in a validated Coping with Humor Scale (McGhee's SHS was not administered, since the primary concern in the study was coping ability). In spite of these promising signs of a real benefit from the Program, depression levels among the patients were not reduced. So while a short-term mood improvement did occur within sessions, this did not carry through from one meeting to the next or to the end of the Program. Since the SHS was not administered in this study, it is difficult to know whether these depressed patients really did make progress in developing the foundation skills assumed (by McGhee) to be required to use humor to cope with stress. If they failed to do so, this might account for the failure of the mood improvement to be maintained.

A major limitation of this study is that it had no control group who received the same medication and therapy treatments this group did—but lacked the humor intervention. So it is always possible that the lasting boost in cheerfulness and drop in seriousness was, at least in part, really due to the medication or other therapeutic procedures that were administered. Since the mood improvement within each session was clearly due to the humor activities and discussion within the session, future research may still show that real internalization of the habits and skills composing the 7HH Program can generate a lasting improvement in the mood of depressed patients.

It should be noted that these patients were very positive about the Humor Habits Program, and were quite "willing to pursue the training until the end." This points to the value of conducting this kind of research with a larger sample of depressed individuals.

Reliability and Validity Assessments

Factor analyses of an early version of McGhee's Sense of Humor Scale using both an American and German sample demonstrated that the key skills associated with the steps did form a single homologous factor.17 And total SHS scores loaded highly on the same factor as other established sense of humor scales. The well-known humor researcher Willibald Ruch, at the University of Zurich, refers to this factor as trait cheerfulness.18 The SHS showed high convergent validity with the State Trait Cheerfulness Index scales, correlating .85 with a measure of trait cheerfulness. Separate factors labeled "good vs. bad mood" and "playfulness vs. seriousness" were also found in connection with subscales designed to measure "playful vs. serious attitude" and "positive vs. negative mood."

This same study found internal reliability coefficients of .92 and .90 for the total SHS scores in the US and German sample, respectively, using the previous version of the SHS. Reliability coefficients of the six subscales (with 5 items each) ranged from .56 (for laughter) to .78, with a median of .71. Only the laughter subscale failed to meet the .60 threshold typically considered the lower bound of acceptable reliability for research purposes. Factor structure data are not yet available for the final version of the scale (which contained four, instead of five, items for each subscale). The Australian study, however, used the new version of the SHS scale and found a reliability coefficient of .95 for the total SHS, with reliabilities for the six subscales ranging from .72 to .93.

Appendix 2

Teaching the 7 Humor Habits Program as Part of a College Course

Over the past decade a growing number of college courses have included completion of the 7 Humor Habits Program as part of a broader set of requirements for a course focusing on humor research. Each instructor adapts the Program to the course as s/he sees fit. My impression is that while students do typically take the pre- and post-tests in these courses, the test results are generally for the students own personal use and benefit. They are generally not used for any research purpose. One exception to this pattern has been the efforts of Dr. William Andress, at LaSierra University (and formerly at my *alma mater*, Oakland University, in Michigan). Dr. Andress has offered numerous courses focusing on humor and health (he generally calls his course "Laughter Therapy") which included completion of the SHHP. He has obtained data on the effectiveness of the Program using college students. Some of his findings are discussed in the previous section.

Dr. Andress finds that a course including the 7HH Program works best with a semester system, but can also work with a quarter system. It also works best as a 4-hour course, meeting twice a week (e.g., Tuesday and Thursday schedule. Tuesday is devoted to a discussion of general research and theoretical issues, while Thursday focuses on the Humor Habits Program. The SHS pre-test is administered the first week of class, and the following eight weeks are devoted to the Program itself. This takes the instructor up to the 9th week; the last week (quarter system) or six weeks (semester system) are devoted to any other supporting materials the instructor chooses. In the case of a semester system, the post-test is best administered the week after completion of the Program, so as to avoid the influence of the added stress of papers and final exams.

Students are assigned Humor Log exercises and Home Play activities each Thursday. The first half of the following Thursday is then used to discuss the Home Play and exercises assigned for the previous week. (Only a small selection of the exercises and Home Play activities are assigned so as to make the course assignments manageable.) Some humor exercises are practiced in the class itself.

Students are asked to bring some kind of humor or laughter activity to start each Thursday class. They are then broken into small groups to discuss with each other what they did to build the humor habit they were working on for that week. Some students are then asked to share their experience from the previous week in front of the whole class. The final hour is spent discussing issues and activities related to the Humor Habit to be worked on in the coming week. All students keep track of the activities in which they engage during the week in a Humor Diary.

In addition to completing the SHS post-test upon completion of the program, Dr. Andress also asks his students to do a more open-ended self-evaluation of the impact of the 7HH Program upon them.

Dr. Andress' students are often initially disappointed that the course is a "serious" course, and that they have to study substantive content. They are typically expecting some kind of "comedy show." But, he added, "They quickly warm up to the class and never find it a waste of time." In fact, the course became one of the more popular courses on campus once it was offered a couple of times. Still, many students have a hard time understanding the idea that developing strong humor habits and skills does not mean you're learning to become a comedian all the time.

Dr. Andress has very kindly expressed his willingness to share his course syllabus with anyone considering offering a college course which includes participation in the 7HH Program. This will make it easier for you to launch your first effort at offering a comparable course of your own. His e-mail address is included in reference 1 for Appendix 2.

Appendix 3

Assessing Your Progress in Boosting Your Humor Habits/Skills

The pre-test of your attitude, mood, and sense of humor will provide you with 1) a good picture of your present sense of humor, including its strengths and weaknesses, 2) a basis for determining what aspects of your sense of humor you want to target for special effort, and 3) a "base line" for comparison with the post-test, so that you can determine how much you've gained by completing this Humor Habits Training Program.

A separate test if your attitude (playful vs. serious) and mood (positive vs. negative) is provided, because your daily attitude and mood influence how easy it is to use your sense of humor when you need a good laugh. Once you've completed the pre-test, do not look at your answers until you've completed the 7HH Program and the post-test.

Peer/Spouse Rating

In addition to completing the pre-test yourself, ask two (or more) other people who know you well to rate your sense of humor using the same pre-test. Make photocopies of the pre-test and ask them to simply substitute your name where it says "I." You should be aware that there is a tendency for friends or colleagues to give you ratings that are higher than the way they actually perceive you. Mention this tendency to them, and ask them to rate you as honestly as possible. Otherwise, the information you get will be of little use to you. You should also be careful to rate yourself as honestly as possible. No one else will see your ratings, so rate yourself as you really are—not as you'd like to be.

Having other people rate you will give you a better picture of your current sense of humor. You'll be surprised to see that others may have a very different perception of your sense of humor than you do. Again, you can use this information to select specific steps of the program for extra attention.

One of the raters should be someone you work with—but make sure it's someone who will feel comfortable about rating you honestly. This should also be someone by whom you will not be offended if s/he rates you in a way that does not match your own view of yourself. If possible have two different people at work rate you.

If you are married, ask your spouse to rate you. If his/her ratings differ from yours, be careful not to allow this to generate discord. Use the differences as a starting point for a discussion of why s/he sees you differently than you see yourself.

Pre-Test and Post-Test

Use a photocopy of the Sense of Humor measures to take the test. Use the 7-point scale provided below each question to answer that question. In the space to the left of each item, indicate the extent to which you agree with the statement by writing a 1, 2, 3, etc. in that space. Avoid the tendency to give what you consider a "good" answer. Be honest.

The post-test is identical to the pre-test. (Again, use photocopies of the test.) It should be completed only after you've finished the entire 7 Humor Habits Program. Use the past few weeks as the basis for determining your rating of each item this time. Do not look at your pre-test answers before completing the post-test. You may notice a tendency to try to remember how you rated each item the first time, so that you can be sure to mark it a little higher this time. Doing this will simply make it more difficult to see how much progress you've made. So you should again rate yourself as honestly as you can.

Playful / Serious Attitude

_____ 1. I am in a serious frame of mind most of the time.

1	2	3	4	5	6	7
Strongly Agree		Mildly Agree		Mildly Disagree		Strongly Disagree

_____ 2. I am a very spontaneous person.

1	2	3	4	5	6	7
Strongly Disagree		Mildly Disagree		Mildly Agree		Strongly Agree

_____ 3. I think it's important to always adopt a serious demeanor at work.

1	2	3	4	5	6	7
Strongly Agree		Mildly Agree		Mildly Disagree		Strongly Disagree

_____ 4. I have a lot of fun in my life.

1	2	3	4	5	6	7
Strongly Disagree		Mildly Disagree		Mildly Agree		Strongly Agree

_____ 5. I prefer friends who are generally pretty serious.

1	2	3	4	5	6	7
Strongly Agree		Mildly Agree		Mildly Disagree		Strongly Disagree

_____ 6. I prefer spending time with people who are good at what they do, but know how to have fun and enjoy life.

1	2	3	4	5	6	7
Strongly Disagree		Mildly Disagree		Mildly Agree		Strongly Agree

_____ 7. I get annoyed by people who are playful at work.

1	2	3	4	5	6	7
Strongly Agree		Mildly Agree		Mildly Disagree		Strongly Disagree

_____ 8. I often adopt a playful attitude in everyday life.

1	2	3	4	5	6	7
Strongly Disagree		Mildly Disagree		Mildly Agree		Strongly Agree

_____ Total PSA score (add items 1- 8)

Positive / Negative Mood

____ 1. I would describe my current outlook on life as

1	2	3	4	5	6	7
Very Pessimistic		Pessimistic		Optimistic		Very Optimistic

____ 2. These days, my typical mood is

1	2	3	4	5	6	7
Very Negative		Negative		Positive		Very Positive

____ 3. These days, I am generally

1	2	3	4	5	6	7
Very Sad		Sad		Happy		Very Happy

____ 4. I have a lot of joy in my life.

1	2	3	4	5	6	7
Strongly Disagree		Mildly Disagree		Mildly Agree		Strongly Agree

____ 5. I often get very frustrated on my job.

1	2	3	4	5	6	7
Strongly Agree		Mildly Agree		Mildly Disagree		Strongly Disagree

____ 6. I am often depressed.

1	2	3	4	5	6	7
Strongly Agree		Mildly Agree		Mildly Disagree		Strongly Disagree

____7. I am often anxious.

1	2	3	4	5	6	7
Strongly Agree		Mildly Agree		Mildly Disagree		Strongly Disagree

____ 8. I am often angry.

1	2	3	4	5	6	7
Strongly Agree		Mildly Agree		Mildly Disagree		Strongly Disagree

____ Total PNM score (add items 1- 8)

Sense of Humor Scale

Use the 7-point scale provided here to answer the rest of the items below. Again, avoid the tendency to give what you consider a "good" answer.

1	2	3	4	5	6	7
Strongly Disagree		Mildly Disagree		Mildly Agree		Strongly Agree

Enjoyment of Humor

_____ 1. I generally look for sit coms or other funny programs to watch on TV.

_____ 2. When I pick up magazines, I generally look at the cartoons in them first.

_____ 3. When I go to the movies, my preference is generally to see a good comedy.

_____ 4. It is important for me to have a lot of humor in my life.

_____ Total EH score (add items 1- 4)

Laughter

_____ 5. I have a good belly laugh many times each day.

_____ 6. I have a heartier, more robust laugh than most people.

_____ 7. I feel comfortable laughing, even when others aren't.

_____ 8. One or both of my parents laughed a lot when I was growing up.

_____ Total L score (add items 5 - 8)

Verbal Humor

_____ 9. I often tell jokes.

_____ 10. I often tell funny stories.

_____ 11. I often create my own spontaneous puns.

_____ 12. I often make other spontaneous witty remarks (other than 9–11).

_____ Total VH score (add items 9 - 12)

Finding Humor in Everyday Life

_____ 13. I often find humor in things that happen at work.

_____ 14. I often find humor in things that happen at home.

_____ 15. I often find humor in things that happen outside of work & family settings.

_____ 16. I often share with others the funny incidents I observe, or that happen to me.

_____ Total FHEL score (add items 13 - 16)

Laughing at Yourself

_____ 17. I have no trouble poking fun at my physical imperfections.

_____ 18. I often find humor in my own embarrassing incidents or personal blunders.

_____ 19. I often share with others the humor in my blunders/embarrassing incidents.

_____ 20. I find it easy to laugh when I am the butt of the joke.

_____ Total LY score (add items 17 – 20)

Humor Under Stress

_____ 21. My sense of humor rarely abandons me under stress.

_____ 22. I often use my sense of humor to control the effect of stress on my mood.

_____ 23. I often use humor at work to reduce stress and stay effective on the job.

_____ 24. My sense of humor is my most effective tool in coping with life stress.

_____ Total HUS score (add items 21 – 24)

_____ Total Sense of Humor score (add items 1– 24)

This is your Humor Quotient. Lowest possible score = 24. Highest = 168. Your goal should be to score at 140 or higher. For the Playful/Serious Attitude and Positive/Negative Mood Scales, your goal should be to raise your score up to 45 or higher.

REFERENCES

The Third Habit

1. Levenson, R.W., et al. (1990). Voluntary facial action generates emotion-specific autonomic system activity. *Psychophysiol.*, 27, 363-384.
2. Santibanez, H. & Block, S. (1986). A qualitative analysis of emotional effector patterns and their feedback. *Pavlovian J. of Biol. Sci.*, 21, 108-116.

The Fourth Habit

1. Muller, R. (1988). *The World Joke Book.* New York: Amity House.

The Fifth Habit

1. John, G. (1993). The warmth of the unlikely. *Christian Science Monitor*, Aug. 6, p. 16.

The Seventh Habit

1. Bombeck, E. (1989). *I want to Grow Up, I Want to Grow Hair, I Want to Go to Boise.* New York: Harper & Row.

Appendix 1

1. Gunderson, A.L. (1998). A comparison of the effect of two humor programs on self-reported coping capabilities and pain among the elderly. Unpublished Master's Thesis, Montclair State Univ.
2. Sassenrath, S. (2001). Humor und lachen als stressbewaltigungsstrategie. Unpublished Masters Thesis, Univ. of Vienna, Austria.
3. Martin, R.A. (1996). The situational humor response questionnaire (SHRQ) and coping humor scale: A decade of research findings. *Humor: Int. J. of Humor Res.*, 9(3/4), 251-272.
4. Rusch, S. & Stolz, H. (2009). Ist sinn fur humor lernbar? Eine anwendung und evaluation des 8 Stupfen Programs (McGhee, 1999). Can a sense of humor be learned? An application and evaluation of the 8-Step Program (McGhee, 1999). Unpublished Masters Thesis, Univ. of Zurich, Switzerland.

5. Crawford, S. (2009). Humor skills enhancement: A positive approach to emotional well-being. Unpublished Doctoral Dissert., James Cook Univ., North Queensland, Australia.

6. Martin, R.A., et al. (2003). Individual differences in uses of humor and their relationship to psychological well-being: Development of the humor styles questionnaire. *J. of Res. in Pers.*, 37, 48-75.

7. Watson, D., et al. (1988). Development and validation of brief measures of positive and negative affect. The PANAS scales. *J. of Pers. & Soc. Psychol.*, 54, 1063-1070.

8. Schwarzer, R. (Ed.) (1992). *Self-Efficacy: Thought Control of Action*. Washington, DC: Hemisphere.

9. Pallant, J.F. (2000). Development and validation of a scale to measure perceived control of internal states. *J. of Pers. Assessment*, 75(2), 308-337.

10. Cohen, S., et al. (1983). A global measure of perceived stress. *J. of Health & Soc. Beh.*, 24, 385-396.

11. Lovibond, S.H. & Lovibond, P.F. (1995). *Manual for the Depression Anxiety Stress Scales* (2nd ed.). Sydney: Psychology Foundation.

12. Weber, M.A. (2006). Ernsthaft Humorvoll: Humor in der Sozialen Arbeit. Diplomarbeit zur Abschlussprufung als Dipl. Sozialpadagogin. Wurzburg University.

13. Andress, W. A. (2010). Empirical evidence for therapeutic laughter courses on a university campus. Paper presented at the Conference of the National Wellness Institute, Stevens Point, WI.

14. Danzer, A.J., et al. (1990). Effect of exposure to humorous stimuli on induced depression. *Psych. Rep.*, 66, 1027-1036.

Deaner, S.L. & McConatha, J.T. (1993). The relation of humor to depression and personality. *Psych. Rep.*, 72, 755-763.

Nezu, A.M., et al. (1988). Sense of humor as a moderator of the relation between stressful events and psychological distress: A prospective analysis. *J. of Pers. & Soc. Psych.*, 54, 520-525.

15. Wilbers, J. (2009). Humour appreciation and emotion regulation: Training humour abilities in depressive patients. Masters Thesis, Maastricht University, Germany.

16. Falkenberg, I., et al. (Submitted for publication). Implementation of a manual-based training of humor abilities in patients with depression: A pilot study.

17. Ruch, W. & Carrell, A.T. (1998). Trait cheerfulness and the sense of humor. *Pers. & Indiv. Diffs.*, 24, 551-558.

18. Ruch, W. & Kohler, G. (1998). A temperament approach to humor. In W. Ruch (Ed.), *The Sense of Humor: Explorations of a Personality Characteristic*. New York: Mouton de Gruyter, pp. 203-228.

Appendix 2

1. To contact Dr. William Andress at LaSierra University for a copy of his course syllabus on Laughter Therapy (which includes a description of how he uses the 7 Humor Habits Program, e-mail him at <u>wandress@lasierra.edu</u>.